TERESA SHIEL

SWEET JOURNEY

TO TRANSFORMATION

PRACTICAL STEPS TO LOSE
WEIGHT AND LIVE HEALTHY

Write
THE VISION.NET

Contact the author at: www.TeresaShieldsParker.com

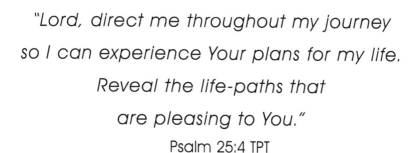

"*Lord, direct me throughout my journey
so I can experience Your plans for my life.
Reveal the life-paths that
are pleasing to You.*"
Psalm 25:4 TPT

DEDICATION

To the thousands of individuals
who have been through
my coaching programs and courses,
you are bold, beautiful and beloved.
The thing that brings me great pleasure
is watching each of you embark on your
own journey to transformation.
The weight loss, of course, is amazing,
but to me the most beautiful part
is when you are able to lay your emotional
baggage at Jesus' feet
and finally embrace all that He has for you.
I am living my destiny dream when I see you
having your own personal transformation!
That truly is the sweetest thing
on this earth.
Sweet Grace for Your Journey!

TESTIMONIES

I started having weight issues after my divorce from my first husband. From Teresa Shields Parker's courses and coaching groups, I received the tools I need to help face everyday life challenges. I have successfully lost 93 pounds and kept it off for over three years.

One big issue I had to resolve was why I could lose weight and then stop whenever someone praised me. Teresa helped me understand that I had a fear of being hurt where men were concerned.

I have lost 93 pounds and have kept it off for three years.

Although I didn't think getting married again was even something I desired, I am now married to a surprise blessing from God in the form of a loving and caring husband.

My husband and I both try to eat healthy and work out. I personally love Crossfit and can now deadlift 225 pounds.. When I started I could barely lift 85 pounds. It feels great to get stronger and I love being in the weightlifting community. We've also taken on challenges such as running a 5K together. Life is always a new adventure. It's not as easy as I thought it would be to stay focused on the things I eat. In a blink of an eye food can become an issue again. The good news is I have all the tools I need to get back on track.

I never dreamed I'd be able to lose weight, keep it off, and feel great!

In addition to losing weight, I learned to forgive deep-seated hurts that I wasn't even aware were an issue in my life until they continued to stop me dead in my tracks.

I am so thankful for God's grace in my life. I now know completely that His love towards me is never-ending. God gives me strength when I am weak and the persistence to keep pushing forward. He is so good!

Teresa has been given a special gift to minister to those of us who have begun to believe that we will never be able to be active again, love again, forgive again, or accept God's outrageous love for us again. I never dreamed I'd be able to lose weight, keep it off, and feel great. With Teresa's help and God's I have.

Michelle Moore, Columbia, MO

DIABETES AND 68 POUNDS GONE

I was diagnosed with diabetes about 18 months ago. I did not take medication, but I got serious about a lifestyle change. I have quit lying to myself and started taking care of me.

I've lost 68 pounds! The diabetes is gone and my A1C was 5.1 for my latest lab. I am off blood pressure medication and currently take no medications. It has been a wonderful year! I'm so grateful that I'm on my way to many, many more great years. As long as I follow what God shows me to do I know the weight will stay gone!

Dawn Wisdom Kinstley, New Braunfels, TX

OUT OF WHEELCHAIR AND 67 POUNDS GONE

I'm a 68 year-old mother and grandmother. I have been overweight my entire adult life. My weight has been a huge obstacle and has led to many other issues, such as health problems. When I first got acquainted with Teresa in 2015 I was mostly wheelchair bound, didn't drive, and was resigned to living a low-level life in my house.

Since I have been in her courses and groups I have lost 67 pounds, am out of my wheelchair, back to driving, and now am able to work as a volunteer. My weight loss has been slow and steady, but the pounds are coming off and staying off.

> I know with God's help I am not only changing, I am transforming.

When I first started this journey I was afraid I was too old and too far gone to change. I know with God's help I am not only changing, I am transforming. With Teresa's help I now see that God really does care about my healthy living journey.

Peggy Burgess, Northcumberland, PA

AUTHOR'S NOTE

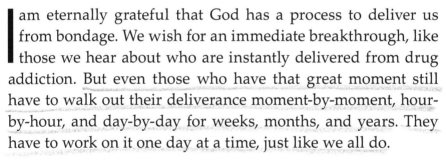

I am eternally grateful that God has a process to deliver us from bondage. We wish for an immediate breakthrough, like those we hear about who are instantly delivered from drug addiction. But even those who have that great moment still have to walk out their deliverance moment-by-moment, hour-by-hour, and day-by-day for weeks, months, and years. They have to work on it one day at a time, just like we all do.

It is absolutely the same with each of us. We have programmed ourselves to self-destruct with the types and quantities of foods we eat. We've done it over a period of years to the point where we don't see that we are setting ourselves up for personal disaster.

To reverse what we've already set in motion, we have to reprogram ourselves for life and not death, for blessings and not curses.[1] We have to change, which is an uncomfortable word to most of us. Change sounds hard. We want easy.

It's a whole lot easier to change a bad behavior that we've only been doing for a month or so, rather than one we've been working on making a core element of our lives for years and years. The great thing, though, is God's help and strength speeds up the process so that 10, 20, 30, even 40 years of bad habits can be changed in a relatively short span of time.

It may take a year to get started and another to solidify the changes. Then, it may take several more to walk through the difficulties and trials life throws at us to really cement our change. Still, it takes less time to change our bad choices than it took to make them something we do automatically without thinking.

QUICK WEIGHT LOSS SCHEMES DON'T WORK

The diet mentality of our culture tells us we can lose all this weight very quickly, which is true. We can, but we will not have changed any habits and will eventually regain the weight we lost, plus more.

Habit change is a process. It's something we have to desire so much that we will work on it every day. We will give up the things that are killing us and begin to add back into our lives things that are life-giving.

It's like getting any kind of college degree. If we really want that diploma we have to be present at every class, pay close attention to assignments, get papers written and turned in on time, and show we know how to apply the lessons taught come test time. Only then do we get the reward of a good grade.

If we are diligent we will pass. If we goof off, go out to eat with our friends whenever we want, skip class, forget what we learned, or don't even show up we know what will happen when the semester grade comes. We don't even have to open the envelope. We know we failed.

If we had just shown up for class and attempted to take the tests, we would probably have passed. Instead, we expected the teacher to have mercy on us and give us a good grade even though we didn't put out any effort. We, however, aren't on our healthy living journey to get a grade. We are on this journey to transform our lives. It's even more imperative that we are committed to the process.

One time my son was ready to drop out of a college class. It wasn't a class he liked, but it was one he needed for his degree. It was also one he had paid for.

> We don't appreciate the things that come easy.

He had a choice. He could drop the course, not get a refund, and not have a failing grade on his transcript. Or he could stay in the class, buckle down, go to study sessions, ask the teacher questions, study for the test, get at least a passing grade, and make the money he spent count for something.

He chose the latter. He wanted to have his money count for something. He just made up his mind that he would put in the hard work and succeed. He was more excited about barely passing that course than getting better grades in easier courses.

We don't appreciate the things that come easy. Easy come, easy go is not just a saying. It's a truth. If it was easy everyone would be doing it and no one would be keeping the billion-dollar weight loss industry in business.

To appreciate and understand how change works, we have to be willing to do the things that seem hard. Giving up sugar and flour felt impossible. However, I decided I was going to have to do what seemed hard if I wanted to lose weight, live longer, have a better quality of life, and fulfill God's destiny dream. Then seeing God do through me what felt impossible became my greatest desire.

The big revelation for me, though, was that God was not mad at me for gaining up to 430 pounds. He was, and still is, madly in love with me. He feels the same way about each one of us. He doesn't expect us to walk this journey alone no matter how big of a mess we feel we've made of our lives. The strength of His grace is there to help us when we feel we can't go on.

> I closed my eyes, stepped into the unknown, and fell right into His arms of grace.

God said, "My grace is always more than enough for you, and My power finds its full expression through your weakness."[2] Then Paul acknowledged, "So I will celebrate my weaknesses, for when I'm weak I sense more deeply the mighty power of Christ living in me."[3] We feel weak in "our human strength, but with God in us we are strong, truly able, truly powerful, truly drawing from God's strength."[4]

By His strength I took that first risky step of faith towards giving up sugar and starting to exercise. It felt like I was stepping off a huge ravine and would surely fall to my death on the rocks at the bottom. Still I knew beyond a shadow of a doubt this scary step was what God wanted me to do. So I closed my eyes, stepped into the unknown, and fell right into His arms of grace.

He carried me through the process of losing more than 250 pounds. Today, He still carries me as I continue to walk out this journey by acting against my addiction to sugar and high-carbohydrate foods.

REBUILDING OUR LIVES

With God's help, I have rebuilt my life. With God's help we can each rebuild our lives. We can rebuild our foundations strong. We can construct our new framework securely. We can make sure the heart of our home is filled with the right things. We can implement the new beautiful design He has in mind for each of us. It is a reconstruction process that resurrects His transformation dream for our lives.

> We have the force living inside us that spoke the universe into being.

We can do this because we have the force living inside us that spoke the universe and everything in it into being. He created everything out of nothing by just the power of His voice. His Spirit raised Christ from the dead. If we have a personal relationship with Jesus, we know that same power lives inside of us.[5]

I spent years wallowing in the world of gaining weight, dieting, losing weight, and then gaining back all the weight plus more. Unfortunately, I repeated this process over and over. During that time I looked for books that would tell me true stories about real people who had a lot of weight to lose, lost the weight, and kept it off. I couldn't find any.

I sometimes wonder if God allowed me to gain up to 430 pounds in order for me to lose the weight so I could share with others, maybe someone like you, how to do the same. To date I've lost more than 250 pounds and kept it off since 2012. In these pages I will share with you the process I went through to do that.

ABOUT THIS BOOK

This book includes five sections, which contain information about each of the five stages of weight loss and healthy living. Don't rush through the chapters. Read, think, and answer the questions. Each chapter builds on the next so that we understand what is involved in this great journey.

Transformation is a progressive change. Many times we quit because we feel like we are failures. When we fail, though, we can learn valuable lessons, especially if we are in a community with others who have our same issues, guided by a coach or mentor who has been there. Of course, it only works if everyone is looking towards God as the ultimate guide. The next chapter will give an overview of the five stages. Subsequent chapters will guide you through the stages.

I want you to understand that this is not an exhaustive resource on how to transform. It is a handbook to get you headed towards transformation.

There is much more to healthy living than is in this book. Check out my website for more information on my courses, coaching opportunities, and more. It's all designed to help you navigate this journey.

QUESTIONS

1. Are you ready to commit to finding out how to begin your transformation journey by not just losing weight but transforming body, soul, and spirit?

Circle one: YES or NO

2. At what level are you committing to going through this book? Circle your response.

- Leave it on the shelf and hope it will motivate me to change.
- Skim through it and read what I want.
- Read the chapters I think relate to me.
- Read the book but skip the questions.
- Read the book and answer the questions.
- Read the book, answer the questions, and implement the strategies.
- Read everything, answer the questions, implement the strategies, and connect with Teresa at https://TeresaShieldsParker.com/JTT.

(ENDNOTES)

1. Deuteronomy 30:19 NIV
2. 2 Corinthians 12:9 TPT
3. 2 Corinthians 12:9 TPT
4. 2 Corinthians 12:10 AMP
5. Romans 8:11 NLT

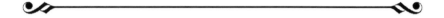

"For I know the plans I have for you," says the Lord. "They are plans for good and not for disaster, to give you a future and a hope."

Jeremiah 29:11 NLT

C O N T E N T S

CORE TRUTH

*"When I am weak in human strength, then
I am strong, truly able, truly powerful,
truly drawing from God's strength."*

2 Corinthians 12:10 AMP

WEIGHT LOSS ISN'T A PIECE OF CAKE

Mamaw was my maternal great-grandmother whom I loved dearly. As one of the oldest great-grandchildren I was privileged to really get to know her by spending coveted overnights at her house.

She'd tell me stories, give me advice, and ask me questions that made me realize she was genuinely interested in my life. She was a quiet, but loving encourager.

I own a large framed print that used to hang in her front room. It's a picture of a matronly woman standing beside a young girl as she sits at a desk with pencil to her mouth, contemplating what she will write.

I love that print because from as early as I can remember I've wanted to be a writer. To me the woman in the picture always represented Mamaw and the girl was me.

When she'd ask me what I wanted to be when I grew up, I'd say, "A writer." She'd say, "Then, write."

That picture hangs in my foyer today. It is a visible reminder of my ancestor's belief in me. It goes beyond just the fact that I am now an author. It goes to the core of who I am.

3

Mamaw believed I could overcome any obstacle to get to my dream. One of those obstacles, however, she unknowingly put smack dab in the middle of my path.

MAMAW'S OATMEAL CAKE

Up until I reached age 50, weight gain was a huge problem for me. Of course, I tried to lose weight by going on diets, but the big issue was the ever-present existence of Mamaw's oatmeal cake.

Her cake was my favorite at any family get-together. A very rich cake, it was filled with both brown and white sugar, butter, eggs, flour, oats, and all kinds of spices including cinnamon. If that wasn't enough, it had a delicious topping that included sugar, butter, cream, coconut, and pecans.

I wanted to eat Mamaw's oatmeal cake and I wanted to lose weight, too.

It's mainly because of that cake that I still love cinnamon and pecans. Thankfully these are some healthier ingredients that I can put in my foods today without adding sugar.

Back in the days when I was super morbidly obese, at least once a year I'd try dieting again. Before I would start any new diet, though, I would bake and eat a giant piece or two of Mamaw's oatmeal cake. The entire time I was on the diet, I would dream of the day when I would reach my weight loss goal and celebrate with another giant piece of Mamaw's oatmeal cake.

Whenever I indulged in a piece of that delicious cake again, the overdose of sugar hit my blood stream and I was gone. I reverted back to eating whatever I wanted, whenever I wanted it. I had no self-control.

I wanted weight loss to be a piece of cake in every sense of that saying. I wanted to lose the weight and never gain it back again, but I also wanted to eat Mamaw's oatmeal cake whenever I wanted. These two desires did not, do not and never will go together, especially when a huge piece of this cake is at least 800 calories.

Still, in the worst way I did want to lose weight. I just wanted to eat my favorite desserts too. Many diets I went on said it was all right to eat just a little sugar. I so wished that was true for me. Even though experience had taught me that it wouldn't work for me, if a diet came out that allowed me to eat a little sugar I'd try it. Needless to say I'd fail every time.

SWEET JOURNEY

I had to realize that diets didn't work. In order to step into transformation, I had to stop dieting. I had proved time and time again that I could never eat just a little of Mamaw's oatmeal cake or any cake, cookie, brownie, or dessert. Eating just a little would be like opening the gate and letting a stampeding herd of wild horses run wild. Once I ate a sugar-laden dessert there was no corralling my desires.

There is a ray of sunlight in my story, though. I have now lost 250 pounds. I lost the weight through a process I call the *Sweet Journey to Transformation*. I call it a sweet journey because for most of us sweet foods are some of the hardest to resist. If it's not sweet foods, then it is foods high in carbohydrates like chips, bread, pasta, potatoes, etc. These foods love to be boss of us.

Maybe our parents told us we couldn't eat so many sweets, but we longed for the time we could make that decision ourselves. Now that we are adults and we can eat as many as we want, we find maybe our parents were right about at least one thing. Too many sweets are too many and cause too many pounds to attach to our bodies. However, we feel like we still don't want to give them up.

> On this journey we get so close to God that we crave His presence rather than the sweets we have allowed to rule our lives.

When we make the choice to curtail or even give up the foods that we have become addicted to, we will find waiting for us an even sweeter journey. That's because this journey results in the very pleasing and satisfying outcome of getting so close to God that we crave His presence rather than the sweets we have allowed to rule our lives.

The *Sweet Journey to Transformation* is really a success path for those who are stuck in the cycle of eat, gain, lose, eat, gain, lose, eat, gain, lose and repeat this process over and over and over again.

In order to break that cycle we need a plan, a way to overcome, a process that will lead us to transformation. This process has to affect every part of us because we are physical, emotional, mental, and spiritual beings. The part we think matters the most, though, is the physical part.

At our core we are spiritual beings. We allow the physical, emotional, and mental parts of us to overtake and overwhelm us. We forget that we are also spiritual. We cannot discount this vital component of us. It is the part we need to be allowing to guide us, mold us, and build our character.

This journey is all about rediscovering the part of us we've buried, covered with food, dismissed, and decided not to pay any attention to. In order to transform we must go through a process that will join all that is us back into one cohesive package.

DEFINING THE PROCESS

For any success path to work it must be in stages that build upon each other. The success path shows us where we are headed and gives us directions about how to get there. It's like a map, but it's not just about pointing the car in the right direction.

It's about experiencing every step of the journey. It is much like a leisurely stroll where we stop by the water's edge, throw rocks in, then wade out, and simply lie back in the water letting the current take us where we need to go.

It's not about trying harder to get every piece right. It's not about beating ourselves up when we wander off the path. It's a given that we are human and there will be a time we venture in the wrong direction. Then it's about learning how to get back on the path when we fall off. It's about how to want to get back on. It's about doing what we've learned to do and doing that consistently.

To define the path, I dissected my own weight loss journey from when I weighed 430 pounds to having lost more than 60 percent of my body weight. Even though I'd still like to lose a few more pounds, I have definitely experienced transformation. I am night and day different from where I was.

> I'm trained in the secret of overcoming all things, whether in fullness or in hunger. And I find that the strength of Christ's explosive power infuses me to conquer every difficulty.

Like the apostle Paul said, "I have learned to be satisfied in any circumstance. I know what it means to lack, and I know what it means to experience overwhelming abundance. For I'm trained in the secret of overcoming all things, whether in fullness or in hunger. And I find that the strength of Christ's explosive power infuses me to conquer every difficulty."[1]

I am content to follow Christ and what He has in store for my life. I can finally say that my life is not my own. I have been bought with a price. I will glorify God in my body.[2]

On my journey I went through five stages of transformation. These stages or steps led me to a place of mastery. Now, I know the process and if at any time I get off the path, I know exactly how and where to get back on. I know this process will do the same for each person who is struggling with the issues of food and weight gain. None of us are perfect, but we can learn how to progressively change.

The five stages are: Wishful Thinker, Willing Owner, Watchful Learner, Wholehearted Traveler and Wise Overcomer. I will give a short overview of each stage to help us understand the importance of each and give us goals to work towards.

STAGE ONE: WISHFUL THINKER

As a Wishful Thinker for at least 30 years, I accepted that I was fat. I'd tell myself, "I'm fat. I probably ought to do something about that, but what I know for sure is I'm fat." I weighed over 300 pounds and more for at least 20 of those years.

I couldn't deny that I needed to lose weight, but I felt I hadn't found the right diet where everything in my life would magically change. I was always looking for the perfect diet that would fix me. I finally stopped trying and just ate whatever I wanted, but I would still dream of what I could do if I lost weight.

Dreaming is important in this stage because it builds the desire for change. I was dreaming of something happening, but I wasn't doing anything to make it happen. When I dreamt I would think about what size I wanted to be. I wanted to fit back into my wedding dress because that was a tangible thing. At one time I had been able to do that. I knew if I'd been there once I could get there again.

This is the stage of acceptance. It's where we all begin. We have to accept we have a problem before we can look for a real solution. We have to know what we need to change before we can change it.

At this stage we are still in a bit of confusion because what we want to happen isn't happening. "I want to do what is good, but I don't. I don't want to do what is wrong, but I do it anyway. Oh, what a miserable person I am. Who will free me from this life that is dominated by sin and death?[3] Thank God! The answer is in Jesus Christ."[4]

STAGE TWO: WILLING OWNER

To move to the next stage, it took me weighing 430 pounds and a doctor telling me that I had five years to live if I didn't lose weight and keep it off.

I still hadn't owned my issue, but the situation I found myself in made me finally want to identify the real issue. I knew it had something to do with God and food, but I didn't want to face what it probably meant.

At the Willing Owner stage is where I identified and owned my issue. To move from this stage, I surrender my issue to God. This is the pivotal key on this journey. Without going through total surrender I would still be super morbidly obese. The truth is without surrender, I might not be here at all.

This is the stage where we must have a light-bulb moment where all of a sudden everything comes together and we see what our problem really is. When God convicts us of that we repent, turn from the issue we just surrendered, and walk towards what God desires for us.

We surrender the foods that we love. We surrender the binges that we go on. We surrender our food addiction to God. We commit to changing our habits. We commit to a forever lifestyle change journey.

A diet will never work again. We know we have to embark on a forever lifestyle change. We have to be willing to allow God to teach us how to change.

We have to be open to change. More than anything, we have to mourn what we have been doing that has brought us to this place. It is where we come to the end of ourselves and surrender everything, especially the foods we live for, to God.

When I clearly saw I was a sugar addict, all the pieces of my life came together like a magnetic puzzle. This deep, experiential knowing inside me brought monumental regret of what I had done to myself and my family. I had to repent. It's the only thing we can do in that situation.

I surrendered sugar to God. I mourned giving it up. It was real. It was substantial. It was a come-to-Jesus moment. It was not a fly-by-night time. It was a deep and profound pivotal life moment. It was a total and complete decision time.

> I surrendered sugar to God. I mourned giving it up. It was real. It was substantial. It was a come-to-Jesus moment. It was not a fly-by-night time. It was a deep and profound privotal life moment.

It's important to understand that we have to completely surrender what we have used that has offended God. Jesus said, "If anyone wishes to follow Me as My disciple, he must deny himself. Set aside selfish interests, and take up his cross daily, expressing a willingness to endure whatever may come and follow Me, believing in Me, conforming to My example in living and if need be, suffering."[5] At that moment, to me suffering meant giving up sugar. I had given up nothing that pulled at my heart more than that. Sad, but true.

STAGE THREE: WATCHFUL LEARNER

Stage three is the Watchful Learner. I had owned my issue and now I wanted to learn how to give it up and walk out my journey. I needed new tools and the disciplines to go on a forever lifestyle change journey.

In this stage we learn:

- How to change a bad habit into a good one.
- How to use SMART goals to tell our brains exactly what we really want to do.
- How to develop our own personal God-given, experience-based plan.
- How to be accountable to ourselves and to God, along with many other great tools.

These tools help us replace the old programming we've set up in our lives that keeps us running to food time and time again when we really aren't physically hungry. The tools we learn at this stage will help us get through temptations and craving and develop solid plans for our journeys.

We will return to these tools time and time again to help us stay focused on our commitment and true God-given desires to follow health in every area of our lives.

The scripture for this stage is discipline-specific because that is the key for walking out our journeys. "All athletes are disciplined in their training. They do it to win a prize that will fade away but we do it for an eternal prize. So I run with purpose in every step. I'm not just shadow boxing. I discipline my body like an athlete, training it to do whatever it should. Otherwise I fear that after preaching to others, I myself might be disqualified."[6]

STAGE FOUR: WHOLEHEARTED TRAVELER

Stage four is the Wholehearted Traveler. It's one thing to learn something. It's another to put it into practice and have experience incorporating it into our regular lives.

This is the stage where we're fully on the journey. We have learned the tools and now we are implementing those tools even when life hands us difficult issues. This is where we fall down and we practice getting back up until we know how to do that. If we know how and don't do it, we know enough to seek help to get us back on track.

> This is where we fall down and practice getting back up until we know how to do that.

This is also where we learn to deal with emotional, mental, and spiritual roots of overeating, along with temptations and cravings. This is where the inner healing journey becomes important.

This stage probably lasts two years or long enough for us to have gone through some stuff and come out staying true to our journey. This is where the trials and tests come our way and we meet them with the ability to hang on to God and go through them. This stage is where we really need a community to support and encourage us when we feel like a failure and to affirm us when have succeeded.

This is also the place where our faith deepens even more as we welcome God to penetrate deep into our souls and spirits to ferret out any existing issues we may not be aware of. It's the place where fear is replaced by total faith and trust in God, who has led and is leading us carefully on this journey.

We are ready for God to put His magnifying glass on us so we can get rid of anything that doesn't need to be there. "Search me, O God, and know my heart, test me and know my anxious thoughts. Point out anything in me that offends You and lead me along the paths of everlasting life."[7]

STAGE FIVE: WISE OVERCOMER

Stage five is the Wise Overcomer, the stage of mastery. Above mastery is the Master. This stage is as close as we can get to Him in this life.

Mastery denotes the expectation that we have arrived on our journeys. To some extent the Wise Overcomer stage does mean that, but we have to have been on the journey for a long time before we ever reach this place.

We have learned, gone through experiences, and are still walking in our transformation. We have to have made our stop-starts into daily habits. We have to have lost weight and reached our goals. We have to have come to the realization that following God to get us to our transformation means we can do anything with God's help.

We have learned how to listen to and follow what God tells us. We fully know and understand that we are just weak humans hanging on to the almighty arm of God. We know who we are and where we are.

IT'S A DESTINY JOURNEY

Being successful on our journey to transformation is the key to our destiny. I had been on my journey steadily for about four years when God tapped me on the shoulder and said, "Ok you passed the first step. You lost the weight. Now let's see how well you listen to Me." I didn't know how important that obedience step was. He wants us to get to the point where we relax into Him and trust Him for every step.

For me that meant writing books about my journey, coaching and speaking. He called me to write *Sweet Grace: How I Lost 250 Pounds and Stopped Trying to Earn God's Favor*[8] which was published in October of 2013.

When *Sweet Grace* became the number one Christian weight loss memoir on Amazon in January 2014, I began to see this was not just a flash-in-the-pan thing. God was doing something and I better get on board with Him. It has stayed in the number one spot in that category for going on five years, with only a few times of being knocked down to number two. As a first-time, self-published author that status was not deemed possible to the world. Only with God.

> We fully know and understand that we are just weak humans hanging on to the almighty arm of God.

When God called me to coach, it was a really scary time. I was a reluctant coach. I didn't feel like I had all the tools to help folks and I knew I didn't have the technical insights. I didn't even know how to deliver information to others that they might need. From the beginning God told me He would show me.

He has done that with every book I've written, with everything I've needed for the website, and with everything I've needed for my coaching groups and individual sessions. Always at just the right time, He has brought people alongside to help me.

GOD HAS THE STRATEGY

There is no such thing as failure when we are in God. It just doesn't exist. It's merely that as humans we perceive failure as a dead end, but God sees it as a place to begin.

Where we are headed is not just to losing 20, 50, 100, or 200 pounds. God has us on a journey to total transformation.

He already has it mapped out. He knows exactly how we're going to get there. His purposes may not be clear right now, but His strategies are being implemented this very minute in some way, some place with someone.

When we get to the Wise Overcomer stage it doesn't mean the journey is over. Our journey never ends. We stay on the path. We keep listening to God and if we get thrown off for a bit we get back on at the stage where we need to start over or begin again.

The journey will get better, but it never ends. We're on it for life. It is a forever lifestyle change journey. Stepping into our transformation means we are now ready to help others in whatever way God leads us.

We don't graduate from being a Wise Overcomer. We just continue to get closer to God, which gives us more wisdom. We haven't arrived, but we are arriving.

> The only way I can be strong is by drawing from God's strength. If I follow what God wants, He will give me the strength I need to fulfill my destiny.

I have finally learned the only way I can be strong is by drawing from God's strength. If I follow what God wants, He will give me the strength I need to fulfill my destiny. If I am obedient to what I know God desires, He promises to give me the ability, power, and supernatural strength I need to do whatever He wants me to do. His strength will overcome the weaknesses of my humanity.

Paul said, "So I am well-pleased with weaknesses, with insults, with distresses, with persecutions and with difficulties for the sake of Christ. For when I am weak in my human strength then I am strong, truly able, truly powerful, truly drawing from God's strength."[9]

QUESTIONS

1. What stage do you think you are currently in?

2. What do you need to do to move to the next stage of this journey?

3. Why do you want to go on this journey?

4. What are you most afraid will happen on this journey?

5. What are you most looking forward to on this journey?

(ENDNOTES)

1. Philippians 4:11-13 TPT
2. 1 Corinthians 6:19-20 NASB
3. Romans 7:19-24 NLT
4. Romans 7:25 NLT
5. Luke 9:23 AMP
6. 1 Corinthians 9:25-27 NLT
7. Psalm 139: 23-24 NLT
8. Available on Amazon and at TeresaShieldsParker.com
9. 2 Corinthians 12:10 AMP

STAGE ONE

WISHFUL THINKER

"I want to do what is good, but I don't. I don't want to do what is wrong, but I do it anyway. Oh, what a miserable person I am who will free me from this life that is dominated by sin and death? Thank God! The answer is in Jesus Christ."

Romans 7:19, 24-25 NLT

COMMITMENT IS A FIRM FOUNDATION

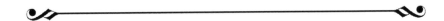

I n weight loss, just as in constructing a house, there is a process we must go through. Even though we may know the concepts of the beginning stages, our experiences are what our journeys will be built on.

Our experiences of going on this journey will become our individual foundations for our personal transformations. Without a firm foundation our buildings can't stand. We must build our foundations strong. They must be laid with the proper materials.

Before today's building methods, masonry foundations made of stones or bricks began with setting the first stone. This was referred to as the foundation stone. All other stones were set in reference to that stone. If it wasn't set properly, the position of the entire structure would be off. This stone is also called the cornerstone.

Jesus is the Chief Cornerstone of the Church.[1] He is the one by which we should position our lives, so our foundation will be true. Our commitment to Christ is our foundation.

He is our Cornerstone. Everything we do is measured by our commitment to Him. That includes our healthy living journey.

STRAIGHT AND TRUE

The cornerstone helps us make sure our foundations are straight and true so when we build our framework the walls connect properly and the roof goes on straight. The foundation, though, has to be strong to stand up to the earth's shifting, rising water levels, and destructive natural and man-made disasters.

The Sermon on the Mount is well known for being Jesus' practical teachings about how to live the Christian life. At the end of that teaching, found in Matthew chapters five through seven, Jesus shares a parable about two builders. One built his house on the solid rock. The other built it on sand. Jesus is using this parable to talk about how we are building our lives. The "words" He mentions refer to everything He had just taught them about living the Christian life.

"These words I speak to you are not incidental additions to your life, homeowner improvements to your standard of living. They are foundational words, words to build a life on. If you work these words into your life, you are like a smart carpenter who built his house on solid rock. Rain poured down, the river flooded, a tornado hit—but nothing moved that house. It was fixed to the rock.

"But if you just use My words in Bible studies and don't work them into your life, you are like a stupid carpenter who built his house on the sandy beach. When a storm rolled in and the waves came up, it collapsed like a house of cards."[2]

This is paramount for us to understand as we embark on our transformation journeys. We cannot get there, wherever there is, unless we allow God to lead us. We may be just wanting a few incidental additions to our lives, a few improvements to spruce up the old cottage, but to Jesus our transformation is way more than that.

It starts with the foundation. If the foundation is built on the wrong thing, the wrong reason, or the wrong purpose we are going to have to tear our house down and start all over. If we don't, some force of nature will come along and do it for us. We cannot build our foundation on unstable desires. We cannot build our foundation on our selfish desires and cravings.

TEARING IT DOWN

I love watching *Good Bones*, a home remodeling show where Mina and Karen purchase old houses for very little money and transform them. They try to salvage the homes if at all possible.

One episode was sad because even though the house they bought was quite large and they knew they were going to have to do some remodeling, they weren't prepared for what they found. The house had been owned by hoarders and had been left full of clothes, food, trash, and junk for years.

The roof, walls, floors, structural beams, siding, and even the foundation were all falling apart. To their dismay they had to tear down the entire structure, including digging up the foundation. They had to start over from the ground up, essentially building a new brand-new structure on a new firm foundation.

They couldn't save this house even though they wanted to. The home revealed great neglect by the former owners. Obviously as hoarders they had tried to save everything of this world. Now that they were gone, everything they had valued as treasure here had decayed and turned to dust.

They had put value in the wrong things, things here on earth that get eaten by moths, corroded by rust, or even stolen by thieves. They had not learned what treasure really means. They had not learned they should stockpile treasure in heaven where it is safe from moth, rust, and burglars. They had not learned that where their treasure resides indicates the place they love the most.[3]

The place they most wanted to be was with the things they felt were their "treasures" on earth. When they left this earth, they couldn't take those things with them. By placing their entire effort on collecting junk they chose their destiny.

REBUILDING OUR LIVES

If this house's story ended there it would be sad indeed. Thanks to Mina and Karen it didn't end there. On that same lot with practically the same footprint, a new stable foundation was poured and a modern home was built with nods to the era in which the original home had been built.

Our lives can be compared to homes. Paul said that our bodies are the temples of the Holy Spirit. He lives within us.[4] God is the owner of our bodies. He paid a tremendous price for us. All He asks is that we take care of the gift He has lent to us.[5]

Sometimes starting over is the best way to make sure we are building our lives on a firm foundation instead of an unstable one. Tearing down our lives all the way to the foundation simply means we allow God to rebuild our faith on the solid rock of Jesus, our Cornerstone. When we go through the process of rebuilding and allowing Him to lead us, we will have lasting change and total transformation.

> **Starting over is the best way to make sure we are building our lives on a firm foundation.**

We will not try to skip steps in the process. We will go from Wishful Thinker to Willing Owner to Watchful Learner to Wholehearted Traveler and then, Wise Overcomer. We move from acceptance that we have a problem, to owning the problem, then acting against our issue by walking out our journeys through discipline and experience. Then, we finally allow the Master to become Master of our journey.

The process must be slow and steady, not rushed and pushed. We must understand and implement each stage before moving to the next. Think of it as building a house. We can't build the framework before we build the foundation. We can't add the design elements to the house until every part of the house is completed. We must rebuild our lives step-by-step, so transformation is firmly set within us. It's only then that we will be changed from the inside out.[6]

At each stage we want not just to learn what the truth is so we can pass a written test, we want to experience God's truth. Jesus was clear about this when He spoke to the Jews who were claiming to believe in Him. He told them, "If you stick with this, living out what I tell you, you are My disciples for sure. Then you will experience for yourselves the truth, and the truth will free you."[7]

No one can take our experiences away from us. People can argue against our knowledge, but what we know in our gut they are real because we have lived through them. Our experiences reside in the deepest part of us and the truths they reveal will be seen in our actions.

If this seems like a hard process it is if we're trying to do it in our own strength. Before I learned this truth I constantly wondered if God would really help me on my journey. After all, I got myself into this mess.

It's not like I was unaware of what I was doing to my body. I was an intelligent woman and successful in other areas. Why couldn't I fix the biggest mess I'd ever made? Why couldn't I lose weight and keep it off? Why after being on every diet imaginable was I sitting there weighing 430 pounds?

God wants us whole and healthy. He will be actively engaged in our lives to bring that to pass if we invite Him to be involved and if we show Him we are committed to following Him. If we're still trying to do it our way and eating whatever we want, He will wait until we are ready.

GOD DOESN'T FORCE US

He won't make us follow Him. He wants us to follow, but He allows us to make that choice. If we are committed to Him and we want Him to show us, He will make the way clear. If we are willing to follow Him, He will help us get to the place where we operate in wholeness, but He will not force us to obey Him. It must be our decision.

God makes everything holy and whole and will do the same for us. He will put us together—spirit, soul, and body—and keep us fit for the coming of our Master, Jesus Christ. He is always faithful to fulfill His promises. He said it and He will do it.[8]

This promise gives us a success path to follow. It tells us that God is the one who will help us get to the end goal. The goal in this life is being with Jesus as a healthy and whole person. We might say, but I'm not that at all. Here's what we don't factor in, though. God says He will take us there. If God wants it for us, we can depend on Him to help us get there. He wants us to be presented blameless in every way. It's not just enough to follow God theologically. We must follow Him in our everyday actions as well.

> The One who called you is completely dependable. If He said it, He'll do it!

We were put here in a body so we can overcome the pull of the flesh. One of our fleshly desires is to eat when we are not physically hungry. This is just one of many passages where God tells us that the most important thing is to depend on Him and not ourselves. To do that we have to be committed to allowing Him to lead us on our journey. We will never get to transformation without being committed to His leadership.

All Jesus is asking us to do is to put Him first over the fattening foods that have become that for which we live. We don't live for Him anymore. We live for the foods we love. I was there one time and I'm so glad He rescued me, dusted me off, set me down, and headed me down the right path.

Back then I felt I would die if I had to give up the foods I loved. That's why I resisted committing to a forever lifestyle change for so long. I thought I would surely be suffering if I couldn't eat what everyone else was eating.

Jesus calls us to a much deeper level of commitment than just getting on track with our food, drink, rest, exercise, and work. We may think we are on another diet, but God has different plans. He wants to use our desire to lose weight to draw us so close to Him that we will be able to listen to and follow His voice no matter what.

He's calling us to be all-in for Him in every area. We're just starting in the one area that's slowly killing us. We have to accept where we are and what the denying our problem is doing to us.

OVERCOMING DENIAL

To be committed to change we have to know what we are changing and how we will know when we've changed. It's a lot like our home remodelers. They had to figure out what they were dealing with and how much had to change before they could begin to either remodel or rebuild the house they were working on.

We must come out of denial. Denial tells us, "You don't need to be that drastic with your plan. Just go on another diet. Problem solved. Why do you need to change anyway? You're alive, aren't you?"

Denial is the devil's playground. If he can get us to deny we have a problem, then we can just keep going farther and farther in the wrong direction. The sooner we stop and recognize where we are, the sooner we will be able to start the process of change.

If we never understand we have a problem we will stay the same. Change comes when the weight of the problem becomes heavier than the desire to stay in our uncomfortable comfort. We must desire change above everything else.

> Change comes when the weight of the problem becomes heavier than the desire to stay in our uncomfortable comfort.

There will come a time when we don't feel like continuing our journey and want to just lay down and die. When those times come we must have made a firm commitment to the process of transformation no matter how hard it may seem.

Years ago, I went through a workshop. I didn't know anything about it except it was too expensive for me at the time. Two friends, who had been through, each told me they'd pay half my way. I was editing and publishing a regional Christian newspaper at the time and I thought since the man running the workshop was my adult Sunday School teacher maybe I'd go and just write an article about it.

I had no personal commitment to change anything about myself. I was there in reporter or observation mode. The first night they had us all standing outside the room. A lot of people who'd been to the seminar before were there along with my friends who invited me. When it was time to begin, the doors opened to a dark room playing some classical symphony with the timpani pounding.

We were told at the door to put our things to the left and take a seat in the circle. Then the trainer began to talk. "We are all here for a reason. Each of us is on a journey. We want something for our lives that will bring us greater freedom. Our journeys will take commitment to the processes we introduce.

"Right now, I want you to think about this next question. How committed are you to this process with zero being no commitment and 10 being wow, I'm all in. I'm 100 percent committed."

Immediately I felt like I was a two. I was there for the show. I wasn't there for anything else. I would stay because my friends paid my fee, but I definitely wasn't there for the next thing he introduced.

BECOMING OPEN

"Let's do some sharing. Stand and share where you are and why."

I enacted observer face and an obstinate sitting position with legs crossed and arms folded. I stared at the floor. Then, to my surprise, people started getting up and sharing. The first ones who stood were the go-getter types. They were all passion and excitement. They were all in, but they had valid reasons why they wanted the process to work for them.

Then one brave woman stood and said she was a two because she was skeptical anything would help her. Yes, someone like me. I greatly identified with her.

"What are the barriers that keep you at a two," the trainer asked her.

I don't remember what she said, but I remember my own silent answer. "I don't want to have to stand up in front of all these strangers and tell them my biggest problem is what they already know just by looking at me. Of course my weight is the barrier that has me stuck and won't let me move forward." I probably was pushing 350 at that time.

Then he asked her, "What would it take to move you to a five?"

My unspoken answer was, "It would take understanding what has been driving me to eat. Actually, that would move me to a 10 if I felt anything at all could help me figure that out. It has to be more than I was just born fat."

> Today I'm a 10. And that's WOW!

When I came back to myself he was asking us another question. "How is this exercise a reflection of how you do your life? What would the result be if you always stayed at a two? What would it be if you could move to a 10?"

He had my wheels turning. I knew if I stayed at a two I'd be stuck for life. If by some chance I could begin to live my life at a 10 I knew I could do anything with God's help. I knew God wanted me to live at that 100 percent commitment level. I certainly was holding back being all-in with Him because of the foods I loved to eat.

That day I began to dream of what it would mean if I was all in, living life at the 100 percent level, and not settling even for 99 percent. I longed to be at a 10, living a wow level of life. By the way, I finally got there.

Today I'm a 10 and that's a WOW!

QUESTIONS

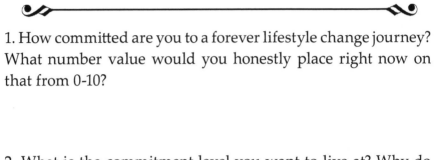

1. How committed are you to a forever lifestyle change journey? What number value would you honestly place right now on that from 0-10?

2. What is the commitment level you want to live at? Why do you want to be at that level?

3. What would it take for you to commit to changing your lifestyle to reach that level?

4. What is keeping you from living at that level?

5. What would it take for you to live at a 10 or all-in, WOW level?

(ENDNOTES)

1. Ephesians 2:20 NIV
2. Matthew 7:24-27 MSG
3. Matthew 6:19-21 MSG
4. 1 Corinthians 6:19 NIV
5. 1 Corinthians 6:20 NIV
6. Romans 12:2 MSG
7. John 8:32 MSG
8. 1 Thessalonians 5:23-24 MSG

CHAPTER 3

MY BODY IS A TEMPLE OF GOD

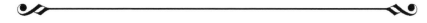

Questions, questions, questions, they seemed to roll around and around in my head when I was super morbidly obese and still gaining weight. Was God mad at me because of what I had done to myself? Would God help me lose weight since clearly gaining weight was my fault?

Would He love me more if I actually lost the weight and kept it off? Did He love me less because I have a huge problem I can't control? Does He still love me even though I've gained weight and greatly compromised my health?

HOW MUCH IS TOO MUCH?

For a long time, I didn't even know what I weighed because I wouldn't let doctors weigh me. When I was asked to weigh, I would say, "I prefer not to." What's even more astounding is that they didn't make me weigh. I didn't realize until years later they didn't make me because their scales stopped at 350 pounds.

There came a day, though, where I was wheeled into the hospital and down to a freight scale. It was just like one of the beginnings scenes from the television show, Extreme Weight Loss. Talk about humiliating. I weighed 430 pounds.

I'd been on tons of diets and had lost and gained weight back many times, but I didn't even know what a BMI was. By the way, that's the body mass index scale that gives a person a number based on their weight and height. Then the BMI chart will show if we are normal, overweight, obese, morbidly obese, or super morbidly obese. It will also show if a person is underweight.

Most online BMI charts stop at morbid obesity. That is defined as a person with a BMI of 40-49.9. Those with BMI's over 50 are classified as super morbidly obese. At 430 pounds, with a height of 5'5" I had a BMI of 71.6. I was super morbidly obese for most of my adult life. The minute I crossed into the 300's I was in that category. There is no category higher.

I definitely weighed too much. To even get to morbid obesity I would have to lose 130 pounds. To get to obesity I'd have to lose 190 pounds and that would just barely get me into that category. It felt impossible.

MY BODY—A TEMPLE?

Guilt and shame really began when I went over the weight of 240 and was considered morbidly obese. It felt like I had wandered into this place where God was disgusted with me. I knew my body was where the Holy Spirit lived, but I wasn't acting like it at all.

It hadn't really registered in my mind that my body, which was a gift from Him, was the temple of the Holy Spirit. It hadn't registered that every time I poured excess carbohydrates, fast food, desserts, and other food I didn't need into my body I was clogging up a sacred place. This body, my body, is the very dwelling place of God's Spirit.

I hadn't grasped the fact that God bought me with a great price, so my body is not mine to do with as I please. God lent it to me in order to have a vessel in which He can live, and I can use to glorify Him.[1]

It was mind-blowing for me to totally grasp the fact that the container in which the real essence of me lives is also the dwelling place of the Holy Spirit. That meant I better clean up my act. I better stop making my body a garbage dump. I need to find out how to really honor God with my body.[2]

> It was mind-blowing for me to totally grasp the fact that the container in which the real essence of me lives is also the dwelling place of the Holy Spirit.

I love home remodeling shows, but I'm really glad I don't have "smell-a-vision" added to my flat screen. I hope that never becomes a thing. Most remodelers carry facemasks when they go to scope out a potential flip because of how disgusting the house smells, especially when they open a refrigerator or freezer that has been sitting for months unplugged with food still in it. The remodelers have to clean up whatever they find left in order to even start imagining what the house could look like when they finish the transformation.

The same is true when God comes to dwell inside us. Before He can transform our bodies to be His sacred place, we have to start cleaning up our lives. We also have to stop adding to the mess we've already created.

THE DEAD COME TO LIFE

Beneath all of the old furniture, smelly appliances, and trash the remodelers many times find mold, rotten floorboards, walls that are falling in, and so much more. The houses could have been in halfway decent shape if they had just been treated like someone really cared about them. When the remodelers get them, though, the houses are literally dying.

The same is true for us. The Holy Spirit desires to dwell inside us and bring life to our mortal bodies.[3] He wants to make what is dead in us live again. When we invite Him to, He will come in with His transformation crew and begin to make our bodies a fit place for His Holy Spirit to dwell.

When I was super morbidly obese I felt like the walking dead most of the time. I needed the Holy Spirit to give me life, but I really wasn't sure if I wanted to do the hard work I knew it would take to make that happen.

I knew enough to know that losing weight took more than just walking through a prayer line and having hundreds of pounds fall off. God would show me what to do, but I was the one who was going to have to take the cookie out of my mouth or not let it get there in the first place.

What this boils down to is the overwhelming, never-ending reckless love of God at work in us. He loves us so much that He gave His only Son to us as a gift. God loves us with a love that never ends no matter what we do to act like ungrateful children. If we have said yes to Jesus we will never perish but have everlasting life just because of His great love.

He didn't send His Son to judge us, but to rescue us. All guilt and condemnation are gone by His grace when we open our hearts and invite Jesus in. We don't have to live in guilt and shame. We can make the decision to follow what God wants us to do.[4]

These paraphrased verses summarize His message to us. It's love born out of grace, which is God's DNA.

SWEET GRACE

I was saved by His sweet grace after stealing candy from the grocery store when I was seven. That entire incident and how my dad handled it by bringing me back and having me confess to the store manager, made me see that I was the sinner the preacher kept yelling about every Sunday night. I was a thief, a candy thief, and I needed salvation.

That night all I was after was fire insurance. I didn't understand the gift of grace that came with that. I understood I had sinned. I understood I got grace for that and forgiveness, but I had no idea of what His sweet grace really was all about.

He knew me before I was born. At the moment of my salvation God looked down through all eternity and saw every instance where, instead of going to Him for comfort, I would go to sugar, desserts, hot rolls, gravies, pastas, and the kinds of foods that made me greatly compromise the health of my body, the dwelling place of God's Spirit.

In that moment He forgave every one of my failures—past, present and future. If we really understood the magnitude of that one act, we would do anything and everything we know He desires us to do.

When my weight became overwhelming to me, God played His trump card and brought me back to my senses. God in His infinite wisdom knew that day in 1960 would not be the last time candy and sweets would get me in trouble.

The odds would be much greater as I got older, but the core issue was the same. I was trying to fill a void in my life with something tangible, like candy. It had become comfort even as early as age seven. It had filled some physical hole that felt like love in some form or another.

That desire for the decadent desserts would only grow throughout my life until I saw sugar as no longer something sweet and innocent, but as a malevolent force out to steal, slaughter, and destroy my very life and thus, my destiny.[5]

RESCUING THE PRODIGAL

God had different plans because His love for me never stopped. He kept pursuing me until He caught me completely. I was His, but in my own way I had become a prodigal. I was squandering His love and soon I saw I was living in a pigpen.

We learn about God's love from our parents. If we have a loving earthly father we are better able to see God as a loving, protective heavenly Father. If we have a mother who comforted and held us as a child, kissed our boo-boos and taught us that failure isn't the end of the world, we will better understand the deep, deep love the Holy Spirit has for us.

I had a wonderful earthly father who helped me understand that Father God loves me, though there was always some question in my mind if God would really love me as much if I messed up. Would He still love me if I started down the road of all the sins I heard about like drinking alcohol, doing drugs, going to wild parties, or being promiscuous?

When I was growing up it seemed there were a lot of things we should do and more that we shouldn't. Although Dad never made me feel I was wrong for overeating, I knew I wasn't following some of the strong words in the Bible, such as "their destiny is destruction, their god is their stomach."[6]

> When we are able to understand the profound power of grace, we will be able to embrace this journey completely. It will become the easiest hard thing we've ever done.

Was God mad at me for eating what I knew was addictive to me, what I had made a stronghold in my life, what I was preferring instead of Him? At times I was convinced He was.

I know in reality, though, God wasn't mad at me and never has been. He's madly in love with me and each of us. He's always wooing us back to Him like a loving father. His grace is unending towards us, forgiving us, and always calling us to follow Him once again.

His grace is strength for us on this journey. When we are able to understand the profound power of grace, we will be able to embrace this journey completely. It will become the easiest hard thing we've ever done.

God knows we can't do this journey on our own. He does not even want us to try. "He said to me, 'My grace is sufficient for you, for my power is made perfect in weakness.' Therefore, I will boast all the more gladly about my weaknesses, so that Christ's power may rest on me. That is why, for Christ's sake, I delight in weaknesses, in insults, in hardships, in persecutions, in difficulties. For when I am weak, then I am strong."[7]

God's grace is power. It is made perfect when we understand we cannot do this journey on our own because we are frail human beings. We must have His strength.

He allows us to continue until we get to the bottom of ourselves. That's the only place we will take our hands off and accept His power completely. It's the place our journey begins.

God doesn't love us more when we do this. His love is so great He wants to provide the strength for us to make it on this journey. His love is beyond anything we can imagine.

LOVE MULTIPLIED

My Grandma was a strong and loving presence in my life as I was growing up. She was my person. When I'd leave her home, I'd always tell her, "Grandma I love you" and give her a kiss and a hug.

Then like a secret I felt we had just between each other she would whisper in my ear, "Oh Honey, if you loved me half as much as I love you, it would be enough."

As a kid, I always wondered if she was telling me I needed to love her more. It used to bother me. When I became a mom,

I got what she was saying. No matter what, there is no way my children can love me more than I love them.

Then I understood. Grandma had love multiplied. She had love for me and each one of her children and grandchildren. It was a love that I felt from the moment I walked in her door.

When she was elderly and frail she'd say to me when I came to visit, "Oh, I love you so much. I'm so glad you came."

A minute or so later I'd look over and she'd be crying. "Why are you crying Grandma?" I'd ask.

"I'm going to be so sad when you leave." She was already dreading my departure.

> If you loved me half as much as I love you. it would be enough.

God's love for us is a love that hurts Him when we leave Him and are wallowing in the ways of the world. God's love for us loves us more than we love ourselves. God's love for us beckons us to learn how to treasure the gift He has given us—that gift of our bodies. Taking care of the physical part of us means honoring God with every single part of us.

When I started my weight loss journey in earnest, I began to see how I was damaging my body in a real way. Even though I thought I was giving myself a "treat" every time I baked brownies, cakes, and cookies, I wasn't. I was killing myself one bite at a time.

I had to learn what it meant to love myself. I hated my body. It had been my nemesis for as long as I could remember. Now it had morphed into monstrous proportions that I couldn't control or stop.

I felt like an actress in some kind of real-life horror movie entitled, *The Blob That Ate Me.* I really didn't feel like I was worth working on, but God whispered softly to me and said, "I love you. I made you. You are not your body. Your soul, the essence of who you are, is led by My Spirit. You are My prize creation. Don't tell Me that I messed up when I made you because I didn't."

> I cannot really love anyone else, even my children, unless I love myself first.

I finally understood that God, as my Creator, gave me my body. I needed to begin loving and caring for it like I did my own children. That was going to take some work. It would take a mindset shift that said my body is not for me to use to fulfill my cravings and desires. My body is God's and I must love and take care of it because it is a gift from Him.

I also had to understand that I cannot really love anyone else, even my children, unless I love myself first. This part of the Great Commandment is integral to our journeys. No one lives in isolation. My destiny and each of our destinies involve people and how we treat them. We are on a love journey, but that must begin with loving ourselves.

"Jesus answered him, 'Love the Lord your God with every passion of your heart, with all the energy of your being, and with every thought that is within you. This is the great and supreme commandment. And the second is like it in importance: 'You must love your friend in the same way you love yourself.'"[8]

Both loving God and loving people is dependent on loving ourselves. We are to love God with every passion of our hearts, all the energy of our beings and every thought that is within us. This means we must first make it a priority for us to have passionate hearts, energetic bodies, and pure thoughts. If we don't have that in place, we cannot love God. We cannot have those attributes if we don't first get ourselves, every part that is us, in order.

The second commandment is like the first. We must love others in that same way. The biggest commitment we can make right now to help ourselves on this change journey is to learn how to love ourselves. That doesn't mean eating whatever we want.

If we were responsible for a child who had type two diabetes that could be controlled by diet, I hope we would do everything in our power to fix healthy meals. I hope we would make sure they got exercise and followed their doctor's plans as exactly as possible. We would do that because we love them.

USE THE WORD NO

We must take care of ourselves in the same way. This will mean setting good priorities and boundaries. It will mean taking an inventory of where we are spending our time and how we can use it better. It will mean saying, "No," to helping others until we are taking care of ourselves. Only then can we say, "Yes," if God says, "Yes."

When I started my transformation journey, I got out of everything I was in—volunteer jobs, boards of directors, doing everything for everybody, and taking no time or payment for myself.

Instead, I started working on myself. I filled my time planning healthy meals; going to the store to buy fresh fruits and veggies; exercising every day; going to doctors, trainers, and specialists to get all my medical issues sorted out; and making my time with God a priority. I arranged my schedule so I wasn't overworking and I was getting proper rest and relaxation.

> I had been telling myself I didn't have time to get healthy. Finally, I realized I didn't have time not to.

I had been telling myself I didn't have time to get healthy. Finally, I realized I didn't have time not to. I had to make time. I had to choose myself first. This wasn't being self-centered. This was following what God asked me to do in order to make my health my priority. If we don't make our health a priority, no one else will.

I began repeating affirmations God had given me. I started with the one hardest for me to believe. I am beautiful. I began repeating it to myself 10 times a day looking in the mirror. Then I added more. I am beloved. I am His. I am a daughter of the King. I am redeemed. I am enough. I am a whole, healthy, happy woman.

I stood in front of the mirror without clothes. I looked at myself through my eyes. I saw how huge I was. I saw the rolls of fat. I saw how I looked at myself in disgust. I saw how I did not love myself. It made me sad.

Then I closed my eyes and asked God to open them t myself like He sees me. I opened them again and for the first time I saw what He saw. I saw a woman with a heart willing to follow Him. I saw the potential He had placed in me. I saw the mountains of weight He could move off of me if I stopped trying to do everything in my own strength and simply let Him lead me. I saw the dreams He was speaking over me.

I wept as I wrote down what He was singing over me and the destiny He wanted me to carry. "My child, I have plans for your life, but they will never be realized until you allow Me to lead you to total health.

"Know that I love you and would never lead you to do something that is impossible. What I'm asking you to do is very possible with My strength leading you. Let Me do that. Let Me lead you."

That very day this scripture became real to me as I could hear Him singing His promises over me. "The Lord your God is with you. His power gives you victory. The Lord will take delight in you, and in His love, He will give you new life. He will sing and be joyful over you."[9]

> The Lord your God is with you. His power gives you victory. The Lord will take delight in you, and in His love, He will give you new life. He will sing and be joyful over you.

QUESTIONS

1. What are three things you need to do to love and take care of yourself better? List them.

    1.

    2.

    3.

2. What are three good boundaries you need to set for yourself? List them.

    1.

    2.

    3.

3. Zephaniah 3:17-18 tells us that God will sing and be joyful over us. What is the song God is singing over you right now? Write that down. Make that your anthem so that when you listen to it you remember how madly God loves you.

4. What are three activities you need to stop? What are three activities you need to start? List them. Note: This is not about adding activities to an already active schedule.

STOP   **START**

1.   1.

2.   2.

3.   3.

5. What are at least three affirmations you will make for your life. To help you begin, I've compiled 77 Affirmations. Download them here: https://teresashieldsparker.com/teresas-77-affirmations/. List the ones you will be speaking over yourself daily. They don't have to be from this list. Choose one of these or another.

1.

2.

3.

(ENDNOTES)

1. 1 Corinthians 6:19-20 NASB
2. 1 Corinthians 6:20 NASB
3. Romans 8:11 NASB
4. John 3:16-18 paraphrased by Teresa Parker
5. John 10:10 TPT
6. Philippians 3:19 NIV
7. 2 Corinthians 12:9-10 NIV
8. Matthew 22:37-29 TPT
9. Zephaniah 3:17-18 NKJV

CHAPTER 4

DREAMS DO COME TRUE

"Where there is no vision the people perish,"[1] Solomon said. Living out our vision or dream is vital to living a life of purpose. It's more important than anything on our weight loss and lifestyle change journey. We have to have a vision for where we are going.

Vision is what keeps us on track. It's what helps us focus. It helps us to soar on wings of eagles instead of just plodding through our days. Vision gives us purpose. Without it we perish, we lose self-control,[2] we run wild,[3] we get out of control,[4] we cast off restraint,[5] and we quickly wander away.[6]

This wording from *The Message*, though, makes the most sense to me. "If people can't see what God is doing, they stumble all over themselves."[7]

I sure know about falling all over myself. I fall easily. It especially happens at night when I get up to go to the bathroom and try to get back to bed. I can't see where I'm going. I have no vision. More than once I have fallen. I find myself on the floor with one leg under me and another at a weird angle. I can't figure out exactly what caused me to fall or how I ended up in the position I did.

This is what happens when the lights are turned off and we don't want to risk turning them on. It's a physical example, but it's also exactly what happens when we have no goal, no dream, or no vision of how we should go forward.

GREATER PURPOSE

The word vision in this verse has been translated various ways: revelation, divine guidance, or prophetic vision. It's really the ability to understand that there is a greater purpose for us than just this present moment, even if that is just to get safely to bed.

We can be assured of this, though, God is up to something in our lives and it is more than just arriving safely. We can either get on board with His plans or stay living in the land of nothing where our only purpose is to get from one necessity to another. The land of nothing is the land of no thing.

We have no thing to which we are headed, except just to eat whatever we want, whenever we want, and however much we want. No direction leaves us spinning our wheels getting nowhere. Sometimes it even feels like we're going backwards. That's where I lived for too many years.

I love this translation of Proverbs 29:18. "When there is no clear prophetic vision, people quickly wander astray, but when you follow the revelation of the word bliss fills your soul."[8] That's what I want. I want heaven's bliss to fill my soul, not all of those foods I used to crave.

God has a vision or a dream for each of us. We are all uniquely designed to fulfill a specific destiny, a different destiny. My destiny is not another's destiny. Even though some of our destinies can be similar, we won't reach the same people. There are enough people for all of us to reach for Jesus. That's why there's no competition in the Kingdom. Everyone needs God in different ways.

There is purpose for our lives. I'm convinced that my purpose was not for me to gain up to 430 pounds. However, since I disobeyed God and did just that, He used my weight gain, and my subsequent weight loss, for His good. It's one of His specialties. He turns our messes into His messages.

FIX ME

In 1999 I was lying in a hospital bed awaiting the results of an angioplasty. A cardiac surgeon thought I needed a mitral valve replacement. Any surgery at my weight was risky, especially open-heart surgery.

I felt so lousy that I was ready for anything external that might fix me and make me feel better. If surgery would do that I was all for it no matter how risky. I thought it might be my magic fix, something that could be done to me that would transform me.

I knew all the negatives. I knew it would be a long recovery, it would hurt, and I might not survive. If it worked and I did survive, I might feel better, be able to exercise, and be able to finally follow a diet. At least those were my reasons, all of which were pretty much wishful thinking.

One thing I knew for sure—I couldn't live like I was. I could barely walk. I could barely breathe. My stomach was pressing against my lungs and it felt like one or the other would surely rupture any minute. I had diabetes, high blood pressure, advanced insomnia, pain in every joint in my legs and hips. I'm sure there were other things that had also been thrown on my medical chart that I wasn't even aware of or have forgotten.

REVELATION OF THE WORST KIND

This was the day the surgeon was going to tell me what kind of operation I needed. I had been waiting all morning when he finally strutted in followed closely by his troupe of nurses, medical students, and residents. They all crowded into my room and peered at me like I was a very big fish in a very small bowl.

The rude, abrupt cardiac surgeon looked at me. There was no compassion in his eyes. He got right to the point. "You don't need open heart surgery. You need to lose at least 100 pounds and keep it off or you'll be dead in five years. Your heart was never designed to pump blood through a body of your size."

Then he turned around and walked out of the room. The resident patted my hand as he left. He was nice. He'd been there before, and I knew he'd come back to process things with me when he could.

Meanwhile my world seemed to come to a screeching halt. Was this it? Was this how my life would end? I could deal with the idea of a surgery that might fix me, but now I was being told that nothing would fix me but losing weight. Losing weight was something I had tried all my life. I knew I co... lose weight fairly easily, but I could never keep it off.

I always went back and started eating my comfort foods. I could never stay away from the delicious foods my extended family cooked. They were like a lifeline of comfort to me.

This was a red-letter day for me, no matter how bad the revelation was and no matter what source it came from. Until a few months before I hadn't had a lot of extreme health issues that I was aware of. In a matter of months they all seemed to converge on me at once. I was 45 and it felt like I was destined to meet my Maker sooner rather than later.

> This was the day I fully accepted the gravity of my issue. I was going to die if I didn't lose weight.

The tangible presence of the Holy Spirit was in my hospital room for the next few hours. He was with me always, but He had to make Himself known to me in order keep me sane in that moment. He wanted me to remember this day. He did that allowing me to lie there in my own reality.

This was the day I fully accepted the gravity of my issue. I was going to die if I didn't lose weight. The words went around, and around, and around in my head. My daughter was nine. In five years, she'd only be 14. My son was 15 and in five years he'd be in college. I knew he would survive. I knew they both would because their dad would take care of them making sure everything was OK.

My mother was already gone. There wasn't a matriarch left for my daughter to follow. She really needed a mother figure. How selfish of me to leave her when I could have avoided this

ly. I saw how my fleshly desires to eat what
wanted, however much I wanted had gotten
ation. I was in the process of eating myself to

I craved that I considered like my friends had
turned the. They had brought me to the lowest point I'd
been in my entire life. It might have been different if I had some
kind of disease that wasn't related to obesity, but I definitely
had done this to myself. How could I even ask people to pray
for me? This was my doing and now it might be my undoing.

CHOOSE LIFE

Sometimes God comforts us. Sometimes He lets us understand
where we have gone wrong and how we can course correct
with His guidance. Sometimes He just calls to mind things we
already know, but have felt were not applicable to us.

A verse I had memorized appeared in my mind. I picked up
my Bible to read it word for word. "Today, I've given you the
choice between life and death, between blessings and curses.
Now I call on heaven and earth to witness the choice you
make. Oh, that you would choose life so that you and your
descendants might live."[9]

I always stopped there, but this day I needed to know if
there was more. As I continued reading words leaped off the
page and into my heart.

"You can make this choice by loving the Lord your God,
obeying Him and committing yourself firmly to Him. This is
the key to your life. And if you love and obey the Lord, you will
live long in the land the Lord swore to give your ancestors."[10]

This was my biblical promise. This was my vision. I wanted to choose life, but I realized it couldn't just be lip service. God had spoken to me through His Word.

The way I can choose life is to love God. In order to love God I have to show Him I love Him. I have to commit myself firmly to Him and obey Him by actually doing what He tells me to do.

Love is the key, but it had to be revealed in my actions. If I follow through with where my committed love for God leads me not only will I live long, but my descendants will as well. My choice of life meant I would have to do more than just say, "I love God." I was going to have to make some serious choices and deep surrenders.

> I was going to have to make some serious choices and deep surrenders.

As I pondered the words I thought about my children, my descendants. I wanted to be present in their lives and see them grow up to do all the things I knew they would do.

I wanted to be present at my daughter's wedding. I even pictured myself there, what that day would mean for her, what it would mean for her future, and what it would mean for the future of our family. I wanted to watch my son become a man, maybe one day even a husband and a father. I wanted to grow old with my husband and go on many more adventures with him.

I knew God wasn't finished with me yet. He had given me dreams and visions. I had more to do, even though in that moment it felt impossible for any of it to come to fruition.

I saw books that I knew were books I would write one day. I didn't know the names of them. I didn't know what they were about, but I knew if I lived they would be written. I saw people who would be impacted in some way by what I wrote.

I had more to do even though in that moment it felt impossible for any of it to come to fruition.

I also saw myself smaller. I'd been through enough weight loss programs to know that it was good to have a dream picture of the size I'd like to be one day. It could be a magazine picture or a picture of me at a smaller size.

Until that moment, I never had a dream picture. Lying there in that hospital bed I saw my wedding picture. It was a time when I'd been happy at the size I was. At that moment it seemed like an impossible dream for me to ever get there, but still that picture was embedded in my mind.

I said to myself, "One day I will be that size again." I didn't tell anybody about it because 250 pounds seemed too big of a mountain to move. How could I lose the weight of two people?

I cried tears of regret. The Holy Spirit was right there with me holding me, comforting me, being near to me, and being real in the time of what felt like my deepest sorrow. I was mourning what I had done to myself and the possibility that I might not be with my family much longer.

I was not grieving what I had done to God or the sin that I had done against Him or how I'd not listened to or followed Him. I was just sad for me.

This was my monumental time of acceptance of what I had done to myself. I even saw glimpses of what the future would be like without me. No doubt my husband would remarry, and my children would call another woman Mom.

Would they remember anything at all good about me or would I just remain a fat blob in their memories? It was really the first time I thought about my legacy. How would people remember me?

GOD DREAMS FOR US

During that time God gave me multiple dreams that I have now seen come true. One of those was probably not such a big deal to anyone else, but it was to me. It was the day that dream of fitting back into my wedding dress came true.

I wasn't planning on trying it on at all. It was nowhere in my mind or the agenda I had for the wedding shower in process at my house. The bride was talking about wearing a dress made by a friend and asking our opinions. A friend had made my wedding dress. So I said, "Let me go get it and show you what my 70s style homemade dress looks like."

Another friend went upstairs with me to help dig it out of the closet. She insisted that I put it on. I said, "No I can't fit into that dress." I was sure it wouldn't fit because I do have a lot of hanging skin on my arms.

Finally I said, "OK, I will try it on and show you it won't fit me." I was shocked that it fit me better that day than it did on my wedding day. My dream size had come true. Another shower attendee snapped my picture of utter joy when I came down the stairs. It's not the best quality picture, but it sure is one of my favorites.

I've lost over 250 pounds. I was present at my daughter's wedding. I am watching my son grown into a fine young man. My husband and I have been married since 1977, have been on many adventures, and are more in love now than ever before. Counting this book, I've written five books and two study guides. Through my books, coaching and speaking, many lives have been transformed.

BROKEN BEAUTIFULLY

The day a rude cardiac surgeon told me I had five years to live was one of the worst and best days of my life. I felt I had pretty much ruined any plans God had to use me. Instead, because of the truth that doctor gave me, God began putting the broken pieces of my life back together to make something beautifully useful.

That day I determined to find a way out of where I was. I hadn't surrendered sugar and other addictive foods to God yet, but I had come to a greater understanding of what I was facing. I was fully in the wishful thinker stage. I was a step closer to full surrender as a willing owner.

Without a rude cardiac surgeon telling me point blank that I was killing myself, I'm not sure I would have ever come face to face with what I really wanted in life. God used him to help save my life.

Today I see that the dreams I had for what it would be like to lose weight were dreams God had for me. They were and still are His prophetic vision for me. Having a vision to guide me on my journey has been instrumental.

It helped me give life to my dreams and think beyond the box I had placed myself in. Could things really be different? Was there a way God would see fit to help me reach the vision I have for myself?

I began to think more positively. Maybe I could lose weight and keep it off. Maybe I could change my mind to obey what God's Spirit was leading me to do. Maybe I could figure out how to deal with my negative emotions in a better way than just running to food.

Maybe I could trust God and actually do what He was showing me to do in regard to my eating habits, my exercise, my work versus overwork, rest, relaxation, and learning how to trust God more than I trust myself.

> Having a vision helped me give life to my dreams and think beyond the box I had placed myself in.

God's promises were what gave me hope then. They continue to speak to me today and will be instrumental to those who dare take this journey. "God can do anything, you know, far more than you could ever imagine or guess or request in your wildest dreams. He does it not by pushing us around, but by working within us. His Spirit deeply and gently working within us."[11]

God dreams bigger than we do. He has this huge over-the-top dream for each of us. More than anything, He wants us to untangle ourselves from the enemy's clutches and grab hold of God's dream just for us.

I finally saw that just maybe, God did have a real plan for me, one He had picked out just for me. "We have become His poetry, a recreated people that will fulfill the destiny that He has given each of us, for we are joined to Jesus, the Anointed One. Even before we were born, God planned in advance our destiny and the good works we would do to fulfill it."[12]

> It's time to dream. Dreams do come true when we submit them entirely to God.

He calls us His masterpieces, His works of art, His poetry. He has a destiny dream for each of us. In much the same way as God puts the design for the butterfly into a caterpillar, God stamps each of us with a unique design and purpose.

We are each destined for life, for beauty, for transformation if we choose to follow after God's visions and dreams for us. Of course, we have a choice. God always gives us a choice. We can choose not to follow Him and what He wants for our lives, but He will always be wooing us, calling us back to Him.

It's when we follow Him in obedience, even in our lifestyle change and weight loss journeys, that we find the deepest satisfaction.

It's time to dream. Dreams do come true when God dreams for us. Dreams do come true when we submit them entirely to God.

QUESTIONS

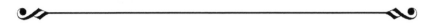

1. If a doctor gave you five years to live today, what would be at least three reasons you would want to make a liar out of him? In other words, what are three reasons you want to live?

1.

2.

3.

2. What is the overall vision or dream God has given you that you would like to accomplish in your life?

3. What is one promise from God you will take as your own dream affirmation?

4. What are at least 10 things that you dream of happening when you lose weight?

1.

2.

3.

4.

5.

6.

7.

8.

9.

10.

5. What legacy do you want to leave? If you were to die today, what would people remember about you? What would you want people to remember about you? Take some time to think through this and journal your responses.

(ENDNOTES)

1. Proverbs 29:18 KJV
2. Proverbs 29:18 ERV
3. Proverbs 29:18 NLT
4. Proverbs 29:18 CEB
5. Proverbs 29:18 NIV
6. Proverbs 29:18 TPT
7. Proverbs 29:18 MSG
8. Proverbs 29:18 TPT
9. Deuteronomy 30:19 NLT
10. Deuteronomy 30:20 NLT
11. Ephesians 3:20 MSG
12. Ephesians 2:10 TPT

WILLING OWNER

"If anyone wishes to follow Me as my disciple, he must deny himself, set aside selfish interests, and take up his cross daily, expressing a willingness to endure whatever may come and follow Me, believing in Me, conforming to My example in living and if need be, suffering."

Luke 9:23 AMP

CHAPTER 5

FRAMEWORK FOR TRANSFORMATION

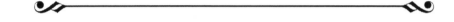

I t had once been a beautiful family home. Mina and Karen bought it for $18,000 from the owners, who had inherited from their grandparents' estate. The owners just wanted to see it brought to life.

The staircase, the entry hall, their grandparents' bedroom, the bedrooms where they stayed when they were children all held memories for them. As did the location, the lot, the back yard, and the trees. It all felt like coming home.

The home indeed had good bones. It had drawn the family together for years, but it had seen better days. It was already beginning to collapse. Mina and Karen could have torn it down, but that's not their style. They believe in restoration and transformation. They believe that homes, like people, carry something special with them—a sense of purpose.

They had to take the house down to the studs, and even then, they had to replace many of those studs. Then they had to reattach the walls to the foundation.

That show really screamed to me about the beginning stages of our journeys. Before we can change anything in our lives we have to have firm unmovable, very secure foundations to support us on this journey. That foundation is our commitment to Christ, the Cornerstone.

One of the next steps, though, is that we have to have our frameworks secured to that foundation. If our frameworks aren't secured they will have to be rebuilt, re-anchored, revamped, and re-attached to the foundation.

> We have to be sure the framework of trust we are building is one that will help us live the life we want to live, one God has designed for us.

If the foundation for transformation is firm commitment to, believing in and relying on Christ, what is the framework we need to build on that foundation? Nothing can be built on our foundations without trust.

In building a house we have to trust that we are building the framework correctly to make sure the house holds together. In our lives we have to be sure the framework of trust we are building is one that will help us live the life we want to live, one God has designed for us.

The definition of trust is a firm belief in the reliability, truth, ability, or strength of someone or something.[1] For many years I was relying on myself to lose weight because that's all I wanted. I wanted to lose weight. I didn't want to change everything.

As such, it took a lot for me to get myself out of the way of my own transformation. I had to understand that a forever lifestyle change is what I needed rather than just a diet. I had to trust that God would show me how to cooperate with Him to make that come to pass.

I had to trust that God's grace is enough and that He is all I need. I had to realize that by myself I cannot change. However, I can do everything God asks me to with the help of Christ who gives me the strength and power.[2]

To trust in God. I have to believe that He loves me. I have to believe that He is a good God and is not out to get me or catch me doing something wrong. I have to believe that He knows what I need to get me out of the mess I am in and will show me how to do that.

> God wants to help me succeed even more than I want to succeed.

I have to believe that He, and He alone, has the power to help me if I listen to Him, follow Him, and obey Him. I have to believe that God wants to help me succeed even more than I want to succeed. I have to believe He really is fighting for me.

There were many times that I was prone to trust in anything I could see, hear, taste, smell, or feel before I trusted in God, whom I could not see. I thought I had it made if I had a good job, money and savings in the bank, house, cars, groceries, health insurance, Social Security, and a retirement plan. I figured if something happened and I went broke I could always trust my friends and family to bail me out.

I knew that it was God who blessed me with all I had, but I was still trusting in myself to acquire what I needed more than I was trusting in God.

I began to understand that God wants me to put Him first in my life. He wants me to put my confidence and trust in Him, all the time, in everything, even in what I eat and how I move. Learning how to rely on God and not myself was a huge lesson I needed to learn.

I trusted myself to get me out of my extreme weight issue. That never worked. It backfired and got me further into bondage to high carbohydrate foods. I wanted to control everything and everyone, but I couldn't seem to even control what I put in my mouth.

> I wanted to have energy, stamina, clarity, and enthusiasm to live my life in abundance until I overflowed.

I had made a mess of my journey, probably like many others who have an issue with weight. I also knew that if left to my own devices, I would make an even bigger mess out of my life. I really had to trust God to help me.

I wanted to have energy, stamina, clarity, and enthusiasm to live my life in abundance until I overflowed.[3] That's a promise from God. The problem is that even though I believed it, many times I didn't really trust God to provide it until I could see it.

Proverbs 3:5-6 is an exceptional promise from God. In this passage He tells us if we will trust Him, the resulting blessing will be shown in our physical bodies.

"Trust God from the bottom of your heart; don't try to figure out everything on your own. Listen for God's voice in everything you do, everywhere you go; He's the one who will keep you on track. Don't assume that you know it all. Run to God! Run from evil! Your body will glow with health; your very bones will vibrate with life!"[4]

If we really dig into what these verses are saying, they will challenge us. I know it's what we need to do, but I also know we trust ourselves much more than we trust God. I found I really didn't want to trust God because I knew what He'd tell me to do and I didn't want to do it.

Accepting that we are the problem is difficult, but trusting that God is the solution makes all the difference. It certainly did for me.

MOVING MOUNTAINS

In 1977 as I was having my devotion time, I read the following: "The disciples came to Jesus privately and said, 'Why could we not drive it (the demon) out?' And He said to them, 'Because of the littleness of your faith; for truly I say to you, if you have faith the size of a mustard seed, you will say to this mountain, 'Move from here to there,' and it will move; and nothing will be impossible to you."[5]

I wrote in my journal, "God, I have a little faith. I also have a mountain of weight on my body." Really, at this time I had gone over 200-pound mark on my scale, but hadn't reached 250 yet. Still, for my height I was close to being obese.

"How can I remove this mountain of weight?" I asked.

He gave me an answer. It wasn't an audible answer, but it was close. It was an answer that spoke loudly to my soul. It was not the answer I wanted and it was not the answer that was anywhere in my mind.

He said, "Stop eating sugar. Eat more meats, fruits and vegetables and stop eating so much bread."

I said, "Nice plan, God. I could lose weight if I did that, but I can't do that."

Due to my I-can-do-this-myself nature, I refused to trust Him. For the next 30 years, I added weight to an extremely faulty and unstable foundation. I was not building a lasting, trustworthy framework anchored to a firm foundation.

What I wanted more than anything when I was trying to lose weight was not just to look good, but also to have my very bones vibrate with life, energy, passion, and purpose.

God promises this outcome in the Proverbs 3:5-6 passage. When we dissect it, we can see it also gives us at least seven scriptural steps to get there.

STEP ONE—TRUST GOD

The first thing we have to do is determine that we will trust God from the bottom of our hearts.[6] Or, as other versions put it, trust the Lord completely.[7]

Back in 1977, I didn't have a little faith. I had no faith or trust in Jesus to lead me in how to lose weight. It was Jesus who was talking to me and I didn't even ask Him how I could do what He told me to do.

I just said, "Nice plan, God. I would lose weight if I did that, but I can't do that." I said that because foods made with flour and/or sugar had become my go to source. When I wanted comfort or protection, I went to desserts and foods I didn't need to eat. When I wanted to drown my sorrows or reward myself, I went to eating more of the foods I loved even though I wasn't physically hungry. I did that because I thought it was filling the emptiness I felt inside.

I knew on my own there was no way I could do what God was asking me to do, but I still didn't ask Him how I could do it. I didn't trust myself to do it. Therefore, I felt He was crazy for even suggesting that I give up sugar in the first place.

Like the stubborn rebel I was, I kept doing the same thing and expecting a different result. I kept eating what I wanted and the Wishful Thinker in me, the one only focused on magic fixes, thought I could turn it around by going on a diet. I wanted a short-term fix for my long-term problem.

No matter how many times I tried this, it didn't work. With every diet and every weight loss plan, even the Christian ones, it still never worked. I had refused to trust God. Instead I trusted myself.

STEP TWO—DON'T TRUST YOURSELF

The first step leads to the second. Don't try to figure out everything on your own,[8] don't ever trust yourself,[9] and don't rely on your own opinions.[10]

I trusted myself more than anything else. I was trying, trying, trying to figure out a solution on my own. I knew it wouldn't work. I cannot trust my own instincts because they will lead me into what I want in the moment. I thought God wanted me to figure out what to do on my own, but what He really wanted for me was to ask Him for help.

My brokenness should always lead me straight to Him. He will let me get to the bottom of myself if that's what it takes. Even when I get there He will keep calling me back to Him. He does the same for all of us.

STEP THREE—PUT GOD FIRST

Each step in this process is logical, but it took me a long time to figure it out. In everything I do I must put God first[11] and with all my heart rely on Him to guide me.[12] In other words, I must listen for God's voice in everything I do and everywhere I go.[13]

I had programmed myself to allow the foods I craved to guide me. They will do that if I let them. I don't have to get to the very bottom of myself before I begin to trust God instead of myself and neither do any of us.

No matter where each of us are right now His hand is extended to us. All we have to do is grab hold and hang on. We only have to be willing, really willing, to put God before everything else. Even if we are not sure how to do that, the willingness to learn is what must come first.

STEP 4—LET GOD LEAD

If we are listening and if it is our supreme intent, God will lead us in every decision we make, keep us on track, direct us, and crown our efforts with success.[14]

When we are committed, really committed to relying on and trusting in God, we will listen and watch for the ways

He guides us and be quick to follow Him. We will ask Him questions and listen for His answers.

He answers us in various ways. Through His Word is one of the most profound. Even if we've read the scriptures a thousand times, there is more there than we can imagine if we read it with our spiritual eyes and ears open.

In any situation I find myself in, God will lead me if I am willing to be open to Him. He leads me through His servants, through music, through books and, of course, through His Word. He speaks to me most, though, when I am intentionally seeking Him in silence and solitude, in a time of prayer and meditation on Him, or when I am prostrate before Him on the floor.

> If I'm not going anywhere, there's no need for God to direct me. If I am on the journey He promises to guide me.

He is always speaking, but sometimes I prefer listening to something or someone else. I have learned I must be intentional about listening for His voice. It helps me trust Him more.

Letting God lead means that I have to be actively walking on my journey. I have to be headed somewhere. Hopefully, it is towards lifestyle change instead of just allowing life to happen to me. If I'm not going anywhere, there is no need for God to direct me. However, if I am on the journey, He promises to guide me.

"If you leave God's paths and go astray, you will hear a voice behind you say, 'No, this is the way. Walk here.'"[15] At the beginning of my lifestyle change journey, I invited Him to speak to me if I made, or was starting to make, a wrong choice.

The way He always speaks to me is soft, kind, and gentle. If I've made a wrong choice His voice says, "What are you doing?" It is like a mentor asking me a question to help me choose a better way, one that is more in keeping with my own dreams for my life.

STEP FIVE—DON'T BE A KNOW-IT-ALL

We cannot assume that we know it all or be so conceited that we are sure of our own wisdom.[16] This kind of attitude leads us to trust in ourselves instead of God.

Self-sufficiency became a way of life for me when I was kid. That was partly because I was in charge of a lot of household chores during my growing up years. This was both good and bad. It helped me learn leadership and organization, but it gave me the false theology that said I can do all things. I was self-sufficient, but I left out I can do all things through Christ.[17] I was acting like I was self-sufficient, but that only happens in His sufficiency.[18]

> I'm only complete when I let God lead.

Embracing this journey meant I had to follow Christ completely. I had to realize this was impossible for me and only possible if I follow Christ. I'm only complete when I let God lead.

This is a big part of trusting God. We have to let Him be the only one we trust to lead us in the right way, the way that is perfect just for us.

STEP SIX—RUN FROM EVIL

When we slip up and make a mistake, we need to run to God and run from evil.[19] We must trust and reverence the Lord and turn our backs on evil.[20] We have to realize that true wisdom comes when we adore Him with undivided devotion and turn our backs on evil.[21]

Unfortunately, many times instead of running to God we run away from Him. We act like Adam and Eve and try to hide from Him. When that happens, we play right into the hands of evil. Hiding from God is one of the worst things we can do to ourselves.

He's always there. He is a good Father waiting with open arms to take us back. Why do we refuse to hand Him our eating issues and problems? Why do we try to fix them all by ourselves?

At the first sign of giving into temptations or cravings or even just going contrary to what we know is God's best for us, we must quickly run to God and admit what we've done. When we do that we are running from evil. We are shunning evil. We are closing the door on what can become death to us.

STEP SEVEN—GLOW WITH HEALTH

After steps one through six, step seven will automatically follow. Our bodies will glow with health and our very bones will vibrate with life.[22] My goal every day is to have my bones vibrate with life. It's not just physical. It's the whole package. It's physical, emotional, mental, and spiritual. It comes from knowing I am right in the center of God's will.

When we fully trust God; when we get our opinions, likes and dislikes out of the way and let God lead us; when we run to God and away from evil any time we fail, He will give us renewed health and vitality.[23] We will find the healing refreshment our bodies and spirits long for.[24]

This really is the precursor to totally owning our issue. We first have to trust God to lead us on our journeys. It is the structure we need to have in place so that we can build lasting transformation. The Willing Owner stage is pivotal in this process. If we don't surrender, if we don't own our issues, there is no way we can transform.

IN MYSELF I TRUST

Our motto in America, which now is quickly fading, is in God we trust. My motto, even though I never stated it this way, was in myself I trust. Trusting myself led to me to trust in many things besides God. These became functional gods in my life, things I relied on instead of God.

I trusted:

1. Overeating to a feeling of being stuffed
2. Overwork
3. Drinking things like both sweetened and unsweetened beverages instead of water
4. Never exercising because I was too busy
5. My career and my husband for provision
6. Possessions like my home, cars, furniture, clothes

7. Volunteering everywhere to make myself feel needed and important

8. Never saying "no" to anyone who wanted me to do something because it made me feel needed

9. My education, abilities and intellect

10. Foods with sugar, flour, or gluten for comfort, stress relief, relief from boredom, reward for working hard, to calm anger and frustration. I trusted those same foods to assuage loneliness, sadness, depression. I also trusted them to give me happiness, pleasure and excitement.

I had to hand each of these to God and trust Him with them. As I handed each thing to God, I asked Him what do You give me in exchange? Here's the list He gave me which relates to each of the things I handed Him. He always gives us perfect gifts.

1. God's Grace Strength

2. His Love

3. Living Water

4. Life until it overflows

5. God's provision

6. His presence

7. The assurance that I am of immeasurable worth to God

8. Self-worth

9. My destiny

10. Father God's protection, comfort of the Holy Spirit and the companionship of Jesus

It's vital that we understand that thing, person, attitude or personal achievement we have been trusting will not lead us to transformation. It is not in anyway a stepping stone to earn God's favor so He will help us magically change.

Change comes when we lay down our self-effort and trust in God completely. The things we have been trusting in are keeping us in bondage. We don't see it that way. We think they are ways we can earn our freedom through self-effort. However, it is our self-effort and the lie that says we can eat whatever we want whenever we want it that has us in bondage. Those two things are against each other and will keep us in constant bondage. We can't do what we want and what we shouldn't at the same time. It just doesn't work.

> Trust may look like a small, innocent word, but it is the framework that keeps our entire transformation journey on track.

What we need and want is total freedom. Paul is really good at explaining why we need freedom and what we must do to stay away from bondage.

"Let me be clear, the Anointed One has set us free, not partially, but wonderfully and completely free. Let us always cherish this truth and stubbornly refuse to go back to the bondage of our past."[25]

We have to trust that God has already set us free and is leading us away from the things which are putting us in bondage. Trust may look like a small word, but it has power. It keeps our entire transformation journey on track.

QUESTIONS

1. What does trust mean to you? Are there areas where you don't trust God? List these. As you write each one ask God, "How can I trust You more in this area?" Write what He says or a scripture that relates.

1.

2.

3.

4.

5.

6.

7.

8.

9.

10.

2. What are some things, situations, relationships, etc., that you rely on or trust in more than God? These would be self-effort types of things that make you feel more secure.

1.

2.

3.

4.

5.

6.

7.

8.

9.

10.

3. Take each of the things you wrote down in question #2 and one at a time hand them to God. After each thing, ask Him, "What do you give me in exchange for this?" Write down what He gives you next to the corresponding number.

1.

2.

3.

4.

5.

6.

7.

8.

9.

10.

(ENDNOTES)

1. "Trust." Dictionary.com, Dictionary.com, www.dictionary.com/browse/trust.
2. Philippians 4:13 TLB
3. John 10:10 TPT
4. Proverbs 3:5-8 MSG
5. Matthew 17:19-20 NASB
6. Proverbs 3:5 MSG
7. Proverbs 3:5 TLB, TPT
8. Proverbs 3:5 MSG
9. Proverbs 3:5 TLB
10. Proverbs 3:5 TPT
11. Proverbs 3:6 TLB
12. Proverbs 3:6 TPT
13. Proverbs 3:6 MSG
14. Proverbs 3:6 TPT, MSG, TLB
15. Isaiah 30:21 TLB
16. Proverbs 3:7 MSG, TLB, TPT
17. Philippians 4:13 NIV
18. Philippians 4:13 AMP
19. Proverbs 3:7 MSG
20. Proverbs 3:7 TLB
21. Proverbs 3:7 TPT
22. Proverbs 3:8 MSG
23. Proverbs 3:8 TLB
24. Proverbs 3:8 TPT
25. Galatians 5:1 TPT

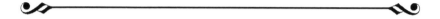

"Now may God, the inspiration and fountain of hope, fill you to overflowing with uncontainable joy and perfect peace as you trust in Him. And may the power of the Holy Spirit continually surround your life with His super-abundance until you radiate with hope!"

Romans 15:13 TPT

CHAPTER 6

DEMO DAY: TIME FOR SURRENDER

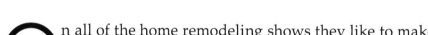

On all of the home remodeling shows they like to make us think they care as much about the house they are remodeling as they would if it was theirs. That just isn't true. If it is our own home where we live every day and raise our family, it will be quite a different story.

When we made the decision to remodel the downstairs area of our home, which included two bedrooms and a family room, we said we wanted to spend as little money as possible. We were just going to paint the paneling, but we first had to pull up the carpet and lay new flooring. Then painted paneling just didn't work with our new floors.

Since it's our house we wanted it done right. We hired someone to rip out the paneling, put up sheetrock, and paint the entire room. Along with that we had them repaint the sad, old brick fireplace to bring it up-to-date and match the color scheme in the room.

Along the way we found issues with windows, baseboards, registers, and lighting fixtures. We installed crown molding to make the room look more attractive. Then, we had to refinish the walls in the bathroom and tear out a couple of closets in the bedroom. These improvements made us realize we needed to repaint everything in the room and walls beside the stairs up to the front hall and the walls along the stairs going up from there. It would have looked only halfway done if we had stopped.

We wanted to remove the stuff that was old and no longer fit with our new design. Of course, we also wanted things that were rotted or constructed wrong to be gone.

We wanted to put in new fixtures that functioned correctly, enhanced the space, and completed the design we envisioned. We didn't just want to make it look pretty. We wanted it to be safe and well-constructed. We wanted it to be transformed into an entirely new space that had a good foundation and substantial framework, and great design

PERSONAL TRANSFORMATION

The same should be true of our bodies. We are instruments in our own transformations. God is the construction engineer. We work with Him to achieve the final product. He directs us so that in the end we wind up exactly where He wants us.

Some of what needs to be demolished to make our bodies function like we've dreamed of may not be anything we thought about when we were wishful thinkers dreaming about losing weight.

We might not have realized that we need to get rid of bad habits, fears, wrong thinking patterns, failure mindsets, avoidance of emotions, lack of faith in God, perfectionist tendencies, and so much more. These things must be discarded before we can hope to become the person we dreamed of and that God intends us to be.

God has a design for our lives far above what we could ever imagine or guess or request in our wildest dreams.[1] He wants us to succeed and prosper. He wants us to be in good physical health. He wants our soul to prosper spiritually.[2] He knows us completely[3] and has plans for our good and not our disaster.[4]

> God is the designer and builder of all things, even us.

He is the designer and builder of all things, even us.[5] We might have many ideas concerning God's plan for our lives, but only the designs of His purpose will succeed in the end.[6]

He's got everything planned and if we veer away from His path for us, He's got a way prepared to get us back on track. It's like one of those awesome movies where it looks like nothing will turn out right and then, all of a sudden, a plot twist happens and it all comes together.

We don't have to worry about the future. God's got that covered. We are convinced that every detail of our lives is continually woven together to fit into God's perfect plan of bringing good into our lives, for we are His lovers who have been called to fulfill His designed purpose.[7]

God has a design for our lives. He is the "Demo Guy." He is the builder. He is the designer. Even when we get off track, He will take those details that don't seem to fit and weave them into a beautiful tapestry that will fulfill His design for us.

If we choose to follow good counsel, divine design will watch over us and understanding will protect us from making poor choices.[8]

Part of the reason I made wrong choices on my journey was that I was not following God's good counsel. I knew what He had told me to do, but I didn't want to do it. I rebelled. All He wants is for us to listen to Him and obey.

God is the ultimate time traveler. He stands outside of time. The reason He knows what will happen to us is He sees where our wrong choices will lead us and where the right ones will get us back on track. He can go 10 or 20 years ahead in my life, so He sees what choices I will make and how they will impact me and all those around me.

There is absolutely nothing God's power cannot accomplish.

It's one of those mysteries we can't understand. This is why complete trust in Him is the framework we must hang everything on. We trust that God knows best because He is all-knowing. There's absolutely nothing His power cannot accomplish. He has infinite understanding of everything.[9]

For us to make the decision to go through the expense, difficulty, and hard work of remodeling we had to have a moment of change. Getting to that point wasn't easy because it involved me deciding to quit taking care of mentally challenged clients in our home.

We'd been doing that for 20 years and garnered a good living, but it also took a lot of time and emotional and physical energy. When I finally realized God was calling me to be all-in with writing, coaching, and speaking, I knew that pivotal moment of change had arrived.

My husband and I decided that if good homes could be found for our clients, we would move them. God answered our prayers and we moved them without concern for their well-being.

That left a family room area with two bedrooms that hadn't been touched in 20 years. Once my husband decided to remove a wall that had created the extra bedroom there was no turning back. Transformation had to happen.

MY MOMENT OF CHANGE

We each need our own personal moment of change for us to make the decision to stop heading down the path that includes eating whatever we want to actually begin surrendering our desires completely to God.

For me that moment of change came when I accompanied a friend to a harmful life patterns group. I didn't go expecting anything to change. I told myself I was going to help my friend.

I knew how to lose weight and at that time I had lost weight, but I also was quickly gaining it back. I needed help and really was at the end of my rope, but I wasn't admitting it to anyone else.

The leader was a 25-year sober alcoholic. That first night he shared his story of how alcoholism had become a major obstacle in his life, why he made the decision to give it up, and how he walked out, and was continuing to walk out, the journey of acting against his addiction.

I was halfway listening because alcohol is not and never has been my problem. My paternal grandfather was an alcoholic and I had promised my dad I would never drink or become addicted. I had kept that promise where alcohol was concerned, but now the speaker was about to rock my world with what he said next.

Out of the blue I heard him say, "Alcohol is one molecule away from sugar. Alcohol is liquid sugar." The second he said those words everything came to a halt in my world. I had a deep inward feeling like a sucker punch to the pit of my stomach. If no one else in that room needed those words I did. It felt like they were from the very mouth of God to my ears.

All the pieces of my life snapped together like a magnetic puzzle. I saw every time in my past when I went on a diet, abstained from eating sugar and bread, and lost 100 pounds. I saw how every time I'd get to goal weight, I'd celebrate and reward myself with one of Mamaw's oatmeal cakes. That would throw me back on the track of eating anything I wanted and gaining back the weight plus more.

> Alcohol is molecule away from sugar. Alcohol is liquid sugar.

I saw myself sitting in my bedroom secretly eating bagsful of candy while my family was downstairs watching television or playing games. I saw how I'd go through fast food drive-ins and get french fries, cheeseburgers, and cherry pies or ice cream after a long day of working. I'd take a drive through the country to eat and de-stress before going home where I'd fix a full meal for my family. While I cooked, I would sample what I was fixing, eat the meal with my family, and eat up any leftovers, especially the dessert.

I also saw how I lived for any event where I knew there'd be great food, including church pot lucks, family dinners, reunions, birthdays, anniversaries and any food-oriented get together.

If I am a sugar addict that means I have to give up sugar.

All of this flashed through my mind in seconds. At the end I realized a basic truth. An alcoholic gets over being an alcoholic by giving up alcohol. I am like an alcoholic only with sugar. If I am a sugar addict that means I have to give up sugar. Then I remembered God said to me in 1977 to stop eating sugar.

Finally, it all made sense. If I had only listened then I could have saved myself so much pain and heartache. Why am I so stubborn?

I didn't hear much else the speaker said, but at the end I asked him, "Can a person be a sugar addict? Is there even such a thing?" This was before I'd heard anything in the news about the dangers of sugar addiction. These days, however, we hear it everywhere.

He answered, "I don't know about all the physical ramifications of sugar's addictive qualities, but I know you can be addicted to anything that controls you."

That cinched it for me. There was no doubt about it. Sugar controlled me. At that moment I knew I was going to have to give up sugar.

I didn't know how it would be possible because sugar was my go-to comfort when I was stressed, frustrated, overwhelmed, angry, ashamed, lonely, overworked, or felt like a failure. I used it as an energizer when I was tired and needed to stay awake to meet a deadline. Sugar was my drug of choice.

COME TO JESUS MOMENT

I left the meeting as quick as I could. I sobbed as I took the back roads home. It felt like when I was seven years old in second grade and my best friend, Becky, told me her dad had taken a new position in church 30 miles away. They were moving in two weeks. I cried for months after she left. Back then 30 miles might as well have been 930 miles. I knew I'd never see her again. I didn't and it hurt a lot.

Thinking about giving up sugar felt as deep as the pain of losing my first very best friend in the world. Sugar had become a companion, a comforter, and a protector to keep me at arm's length from men who seemed a lot like the one who molested me when I was 11. What would I do without sugar?

It had become more than a substance to me. It was as real or even more real to me than any person because it was always there at my beck and call. It was there whenever I needed it because my cabinets were readily stocked with it. I was never without it.

Like a flash a scripture came across my mind. "All things are lawful for me, but not all things are profitable. All things are lawful for me, but I will not be mastered by anything."[10]

Paul could say that, but I couldn't. I had willingly put myself under a different master and it certainly was not the Master.

I had stopped listening to what the Master told me regarding managing food in my life after He told me to stop eating sugar.

"My sheep listen to My voice; I know them, and they follow Me."[11] I had heard His voice. He knew me, but I did not follow Him in what He told me to do.

I clearly saw that I had thumbed my nose at God. I had rebelled against Him. I knew beyond a shadow of a doubt that I had caused Him sorrow. I thought of my own kids and how I would feel if they were following an addictive lifestyle and I tried to show them how to get free.

If they didn't listen to me, I wouldn't be mad at them. I'd be sad. I'd mourn for them. I'd do everything I could to try to get them to turn around. Every time they fell, I'd try to help them back up again without enabling them. I'd want to point them back to the right path.

> God wasn't mad at me. He was sad for me.

I saw how that is exactly what God had done for me. Every time in my life when I'd go on a diet, lose weight, and then gain it back plus more, my God, who is so rich in grace and mercy, would gently call me back again and point me in the right direction. Time and time and time again He never gave up on me. God wasn't mad at me. He was sad for me because of the choices I had made. He graciously rerouted my course to help me get to where I needed to be.

Each time when I'd get to the end of my rope and cry out to Him, He'd give me the same plan. He was so consistent. Right then, I dwelt on the goodness of a God who never gave up on me, who kept calling me back to all that is right and good for every part of me.

Sometime on the drive home I pulled off on the side of a deserted road and cried tears of repentance. I mourned for what I'd done to myself and to my God. I had denied myself nothing. I had followed my own selfish desires. I had made my stomach my god.[12]

That night on the side of that road I surrendered sugar to God. I laid it on the altar. It felt like I cut out my heart and laid it there. In a way that's exactly what I did because sugar had become my passion.

I said, "God I don't know how to do this, but right now I'm telling You that I'm laying sugar at Your feet. I choose You, but I admit I am scared I will mess up again. I don't know how to do this. I want sugar out of my life, but I see it has become a habit, a stronghold, a fortress, and I know it will take work to remove. Still, I lay it down. Show me, teach me how to do this so I stop making an even bigger mess of my life."

> Show me, teach me how to do this so I stop making an even bigger mess of my ife.

When I got home I did what I always do when God and I have had an important encounter. I wrote something to remember the moment. I wrote a story. It's called "Good-Bye Sugar."[13]

The closing says, "This is good-bye. You are no longer my friend. I see you for the monster you are. Sugar, you are out of my life for good. Oh, and don't try coming back. I will not change my mind.

"I know now, I have been putting you above God in my life and above my own desire to live. I will not do that any longer. God is my comforter, companion, and protector. No substance can provide for me like He can. I see you for what you are. You are a tool of the devil in my life.

"I am finally free of you and believe me, nothing tastes as good as freedom feels. Nothing!"

FREEDOM JOURNEY

Today each and everyone one of us stand at a crossroads. For years we have been living from diet to diet, but nothing about our lifestyles has been totally surrendered to God.

I was made new[14] at age seven, but this was the day I was made new again. This experience was so significant to me that it ranks as high as my salvation experience. That's because I was older and giving up sugar and the foods that were making me unhealthy felt like I was ripping my insides out.

I was remorseful for what I'd done, and I asked God to forgive me, but at the same time it felt like the end of an era where I was romping through the fields of life doing what I wanted. Now I was going to have to grow up and get down to business.

What I didn't realize was that it was the beginning of my freedom journey. It was the beginning of not being in the clutches of my cravings. I was living for my false self and my own desires. This day I started living for God and because of that He started teaching me who I really am in Him.

This decision led me to the place I am now, where firm boundaries keep me free to love and follow my Savior with full abandon. I can truly say and mean this: "I will walk with

You in complete freedom, for I seek to follow Your every command."[15]

Without surrender, it is impossible to lose weight and keep it off. Without surrender we will go back to our default food plan of eating whatever we want. This is what we've always done when life throws us a curve ball.

God is trying to help us fit into the design He has for our lives. We must allow Him to show us the way. When we follow God, we make Him happy. He applauds what we are doing.

COMPLETE SURRENDER

Surrender is a lot like a death. It's very difficult to have closure if there's no defining event to mark the passing of a loved one. The same is true of marking the death of using certain foods as coping mechanisms in our lives.

Surrender is a three-step plan.

1. I surrender completely to God the foods or compulsive behaviors that lead me to overeat.
2. I mourn their loss.
3. I repent for what I have done and ask God for forgiveness.

Completely surrendering the things we have made more important than God is what He wants for each of us. I love what Paul tells his protégé, Timothy.

"I remember your sincere and unqualified faith, the surrendering of your entire self to God in Christ with confident trust in His power, wisdom, and goodness."[16]

For his mentor to tell him that had to be a wow moment for Timothy. The grounding center of what Paul said is that Timothy surrendered his entire self to God. I want that to be my purpose. I want to surrender my entire self to God every day, in every way. I hope that we each will make that our purpose.

Complete surrender is the defining, pivotal moment on the journey to transformation. It begins the process of change. Without change things remain the same. Without a time when we have let go of doing things our way and surrendering totally to relying on

God's direction for this process, we will never keep the weight off. We will never have a total lifestyle change. We will still be caught in the dieting cycle of losing, regaining the weight plus more, and starting that all over again.

> **Complete surrender is the defining, pivotal moment on the journey to transformation. It begins the process of change.**

As a Christian weight loss and transformation coach, I have a sense of when individuals will be successful on this journey. It's when they willingly own the fact thay have an issue with food, are willing to surrender it to God, and allow Him to begin directing them on their journeys.

Those who do this will step out of bondage and into God's freedom from food issues. All it takes is a leap of faith where we fall into the arms of an all-loving, all-merciful Heavenly Father. I know because it happened to me and there is no greater freedom than being free from the control of food over my life.

QUESTIONS

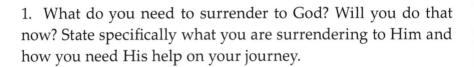

1. What do you need to surrender to God? Will you do that now? State specifically what you are surrendering to Him and how you need His help on your journey.

2. How will you mourn the way you have used these things in your life? How will you mourn the loss of what you are surrendering? Tell God how you are feeling about doing this. Be honest.

3. Are you sorry for what you have done? Tell Him exactly what you are sorry for. Your brain needs to hear it. You need to remember this moment. Write it down so you remember this time.

4. Ask God to forgive you. When you ask for forgiveness it means you have handed this behavior to God completely. Listen to what He tells you or what you sense is happening when He forgives you. For me it was as if a curtain between God and me was thrown open to allow me to be drawn into His close embrace. Write what happened during this time

5. For your closure use this space to write something to mark this time or do something else to remember what your surrender time meant. You might draw a picture to represent how you feel, make a word picture with various words or scriptures that are meaningful, choose a symbol to represent what you did, take a photo, design a plaque with a meaningful scripture or symbol. Journal about what you did and what is meaningful to you.

(ENDNOTES)

1. Ephesians 3:20 MSG
2. 3 John 2 AMP
3. Psalm 139:16 NLT
4. Jeremiah 29:11 NLT
5. Hebrews 3:4 TPT
6. Proverbs 19:21 TPT
7. Romans 8:28 TPT
8. Proverbs 2:11 TPT
9. Psalm 147:5 TPT
10. 1 Corinthians 6:12 NASB
11. John 10:27 NASB
12. Philippians 3:19 NIV
13. Parker, Teresa. "Good-Bye, Sugar.", Teresa Shields Parker, 10 July 2018, tere-sashieldsparker.com/good-bye-sugar-2/.
14. 2 Corinthians 5:17 NKJV
15. Psalm 119:45 TPT
16. 1 Timothy 4:6 AMP

WATCHFUL LEARNER

"All athletes are disciplined in their training. They do it to win a prize that will fade away but we do it for an eternal prize. So I run with purpose in every step. I'm not just shadow boxing. I discipline my body like an athlete, training it to do whatever it should. Otherwise I fear that after preaching to others, I myself might be disqualified."

1 Corinthians 9:25-27 NLT

CHAPTER 7

FOREVER LIFESTYLE CHANGE PLAN

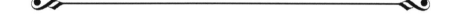

G od has a unique forever lifestyle change plan for each and every person. Developing that plan is a process. It's not an overwhelming process, but it does take some time reflecting on our own journey, understanding what works for us and what doesn't work, and listening to God's heart for us individually.

Before we get there, we have to understand this is night and day different from a diet. A diet is a four-letter word and not a very nice one. Diets and my stubborn rebellion are what propelled me to gain up to 430 pounds.

God had already given me my forever lifestyle change plan, but I didn't want to do it His way. That sounded way too difficult. I wanted easy.

There are diets that sound easy and get weight off quickly, but the weight always comes back and brings more with it. The easy way is not how transformation happens.

We have to ditch our diet mentality and embrace lifestyle change. There is no easy way to transformation, though, because it involves every part of us. What we eat is probably one of the easiest things to figure out.

First, lest we forget, we must go through these basic steps.

- We accept we have an issue and commit to following what God says about our issue
- We build a firm foundation in Him.
- We believe we are worth taking care of ourselves in a healthy way.
- We understand why we want to become healthy.
- We own and surrender our issue to God.
- We learn to trust what God wants for us instead of what we want.

After we have done all this, as a Watchful Learner we are ready to determine and follow God's forever lifestyle change plan designed by Him just for us. There should never be a question if it is the right plan. We know in our hearts, and we follow it with His help and the help of a coach and community. We can work on our own individual plans together because we understand that we are all different and unique, but at the same time we all want to lose weight and change into the person God wants us to be.

NO ONE-SIZE FITS ALL PLAN

There are no one-size fits all diets, although every diet plan out there will make us think it will work perfectly. We are all different. This is one reason no one diet will work for every single person on the planet. It was made for the person who invented it. They lost weight on it and so they decided to sell it to everyone. For some it will work, but for others it fails miserably.

There are some basic facts, however, that will help us understand what healthy foods are. For instance, I've never heard a dietitian say, "Eat all the sugar you want. It's natural. It's good for you." They know too much sugar is too much for anyone.

> A functional god is something we use on an everyday basis in place of what God freely provides.

It's been hard for me to understand that I am wired differently metabolically than say my husband who can and does eat a little bit of sugar and then, stops. For him there is no pull for more.

For me, certain kinds of food became comforting. I learned that from my Grandma, who comforted with lots of starchy foods and desserts. Because I love that kind of comfort so much, I cannot eat sugar today. It is like a drug to me, a very addictive death-giving drug.

As an adult I cooked like Grandma. I needed that food comfort or so I thought. In reality, I had chosen food as my functional god. A functional god is something we use on an everyday basis in place of what God freely provides.

One of the Holy Spirit's free gifts is that He comforts us.[1] I figured that was one job the Holy Spirit didn't have to do for me. He's busy, so I'll just comfort myself with the foods I love. See how nicely I helped God out?

In my lifetime I've been on every diet imaginable, especially all the Christian plans. Every plan likely works for someone, but the only plan that works for me is the plan God shows me and helps me incorporate into my life.

Through the years when I got really desperate and I would cry out to God for how to move my mountain of weight, He would give me my plan. He told me to, "Stop eating sugar. Eat more meats, fruits and vegetables. And stop eating so much bread."

I rebelled against that plan in a big way. I said, "No way. No how." I decided I'd do it my way, not God's. I'd curtail sugar and bread for a little while as long as I was on a diet and then I'd go back to eating it.

Doing it my way resulted in endless years of yo-yo dieting. I can have great willpower for about nine months to a year and lose 100 pounds. That was all I could do in my own strength because after that I would cave and go back to eating sugar and flour,

GOD'S STRENGTH

I am simply a weak human like we all are. Knowing that God's grace is sufficient for me regardless of what situation I am in gets me through. Knowing that His power is being perfected, is fully completed, and shows itself most effectively in my weakness encourages me.[2]

He knew my weaknesses when He gave me my plan, but in my stubbornness I tried to make it happen my way. All along

He wanted me to admit my weakness, especially for sugar and foods made with flour, and allow His power to completely enfold me and dwell in me.[3]

I began to understand that I need to be pleased with my weakness for sugar because it helps me understand how much I need God. If I didn't have a problem that I needed God to help me with, I would still be building my own kingdom rather than His. I accept and fully embrace the fact that when I am weak in human strength, only then am I strong, truly able, truly powerful, truly drawing from God's strength.[4]

> I thought God wanted me to take care of the mess I had made all on my own.

In the past I was always trying to work someone else's plan that sounded good because it offered quick results or allowed me to eat a little sugar or artificial sweeteners. I wasn't trying to rely on God. I thought He wanted me to take care of the mess I had made all on my own.

I wanted Him to just change me so I'd be able to eat sugar and not gain weight. Healthy lifestyle change seemed impossible for me. It looked way too difficult because it meant changing everything in my life.

To God this journey is for one purpose—to get us to the place where we understand our very lives depend on following Him unconditionally. He wants us to get to where we finally walk by faith in Him alone, not ourselves, our abilities, or our intelligence. He's showing us this through our weight loss journeys, but it applies to every challenge we face whether it is finances, career, family, marriage, ministry, or anything else.

In all things we have to walk by faith.[5] Sight left us a long time ago. We don't need to understand all the reasons why. We just need to follow Jesus. We need to know that He knows us, that we hear His voice, and that we need to follow what He shows us to do no matter what that is.[6]

USING FAILURE TO DEVELOP YOUR PLAN

When the moment of surrender came for me, I clearly saw in order for me to live I was going to have to give up sugar. Every diet I'd been on flashed through my mind. I saw how I had lost weight and then regained the weight plus more when I'd start eating sugar again. I saw every one of those diets as a personal failure. I didn't see anything helpful in any of them. My only focus was on that others lost weight on them, but I failed because I was fat again.

Then God began to show me I didn't fail. I did lose weight. I just didn't keep it off. After that I began to look at the diets I had been on in a different way. What elements of those plans actually worked to help me initially lose weight?

One national chain diet was the first diet on which I successfully lost weight. Even though it cost me a lot of money and I lost 100 pounds, I gained it all back plus more after I went off the program.

Still when I had a good job and could afford it, I went back on that diet at least four other times. I always had the same results. I'd lose the weight, celebrate with a sugary treat, and the cycle began again with me gaining the weight back plus more.

I followed God's advice and began looking at my results differently. I began to see what worked and what didn't. The things that worked were not eating sugar and bread, eating a lot of good protein and vegetables, and eating under 1,000 calories a day.

I definitely don't recommend eating that few calories for anyone. It is not sustainable for a lifestyle change that we will follow for the rest of our lives. It only worked for me to initially lose the weight, but we need a plan for life.

What didn't work was starting to eat sugar again, which was the main failure I had with any diet. I didn't engage in any good habits to help change my bad habit of overeating sugar. As a matter of fact, I didn't want to change that habit. I just wanted to lose weight and then go back to eating what I wanted. I didn't want to change the way I ate or moved or didn't move for the rest of my life.

The other big reason it didn't work was that the diet was very restrictive in food choices. To not have any fruits, to limit meats to only one type, and to control the types of vegetables and fruits was too restrictive for me. It wasn't a plan I wanted to, or even could, stay on for the long-haul.

MY PLAN

To understand how to come up with a plan that works for me, I began to write down every diet I could remember being on. Then I wrote down what worked in that diet, even if it partially worked, and what didn't work. I noted what worked best from that particular plan that I could incorporate in a plan that I could stay on for life, a healthy eating plan.

I also thought about what things hadn't work on the diets I'd been on. How could I tweak that to work better for me? In looking over my list of diets, I began to see that eating sugar and desserts never worked for me. I knew my plan had to include cutting out sugar and things made with flour.

Because eating protein throughout the day worked on the diets where I'd lost weight, I incorporated that into my plan. I added in more protein like nuts, seeds, and good protein powders without sugar or sugar substitutes and that use only stevia or monk fruit. From my diet inventory I saw I was not successful on diets that allowed artificial sweeteners, so those were also out for me. The artificial sweeteners mimic sugar and make me crave it all the more.

I had to learn how to find ingredients for, to prepare salads, and to learn to love them. I decided to add fresh fruits and vegetables to my plan. I noted that would mean more trips to the grocery store, but I also knew it would be helpful for everyone in our family.

I had to be dedicated to total lifestyle change—body, soul and spirit. I had to understand there was more to losing weight than just what I ate. However, what I ate or didn't eat would be a big key.

OUR OWN PLANS

In order to develop our own individual forever lifestyle change plans we have to begin to reframe the diets we have marked as failures. Begin to see the positive elements of what did work, even if it was for a short time, and then allow God to reveal adjustments that need to be made.

If something positive comes up over and over again, then that needs to be incorporated in some way into our forever lifestyle change plan.

Remember it's not what we want to eat, it's what is best for us to eat in order to fuel our bodies to make them a fit place for the Holy Spirit to dwell. In my case, I saw that I needed to find a way to give up sugar and starches and incorporate good habits like exercise into my plan.

> It's not what we want to eat, it's what is best for us to eat in order to fuel our bodies to make them a fit place for the Holy Spirit to dwell.

I defined a plan as working if weight was lost initially or if it had an element in it somewhere that in some way worked. It might have been an exercise plan the program recommended, some kind of protein powder that worked, or a recipe that was easy to make and was nutritionally sound. I had to think about these plans in a positive way and separate out what could have worked had other factors been removed.

Those other factors are the reason why the diet didn't work. Was it too restrictive? Did it not teach how to make good choices? Did it not help in learning to manage cravings, temptations, or emotions? Did it allow too much room for failure by allowing or advocating eating a little of the specific things that are very tempting and addictive?

Maybe the plan was too complicated, required looking up foods on a list every meal, necessitated counting points, was too strict about measuring and counting calories, was adamant about following specific recipes for every meal, or even required purchasing the program's prepared meals? Whatever it was, make a note of that and think about how to change our plan to make it work in our situation.

When we understand why we failed we will be better able to figure out what we need to be doing as far as our own personal eating plans.

LET REAL FOOD SURPRISE YOU

Many of us have foods we don't want to even think about eating, such as certain strange-sounding vegetables we avoid at all costs. However, when we develop our plans with God's help, we should leave room to be surprised. Our taste buds will begin to change if we eliminate sugar from our plans. We will begin to really taste the unique and true flavors of real fruits and vegetables and savor meats grilled instead of fried.

I abhorred avocados when I entered into my plan. Once I was adhering to the plan, I began to discover all the nutritional goodness in an avocado. That made me want to try it. Now it's one of my favorite things to add to a salad.

Salad is also one of my mainstays. I used to think salad was a waste of space in my stomach. Then a friend made a salad with pecans, red onions, roma tomatoes, artichoke hearts, avocados, and lettuce. I found adding some grilled chicken made it divine. A great grilled chicken salad with strawberries instead of tomatoes has become my very favorite meal.

Because I listened to God when He said to eat meat, fruits, and vegetables, the salad I've learned to love is in my plan!

We're all eating in some manner right now. Some of us may be on an intentional diet, eating plan, or lifestyle change plan. Right now, what's working and not working about the way we are eating? If weight is being lost why is it being lost? If weight is being gained why is it being gained? Then, adjust when those things are identified.

Consider what else besides food might need to be added to the plan. Think about such things as exercise, drinking more water, resting more, spending time with God, journaling, engaging in restful and pleasurable behaviors like hobbies, listening to music to unwind, and other things that don't include food.

IMPLEMENTING THE PLAN

God will lead us in developing our plans. Understand, though, that completing our own forever lifestyle change plan does not mean we will treat it like a diet and implement it all at once.

This is a plan we implement gradually. It is the plan we are headed towards, not the plan we are going to implement in its entirety tomorrow. We implement that plan by exchanging our bad habits for good habits. We'll go more in depth with how to do that in the next chapter.

When we have gone on a diet in the past we stopped eating the way we've always been eating and started eating an entirely different way overnight. We didn't give ourselves time to develop habit change. We were still longing for the old way we had been eating or living. Change takes time and intentional effort to develop.

If one day we are eating sugar and the next day we aren't, this is a failure waiting to happen. The plan we are implementing should be thought of as a goal. It's where we are headed. It took me several years to implement my plan. It didn't happen instantly. No lasting change ever does.

Today I have certain non-negotiables, such as no sugar and no gluten. However getting to that place took time. Now, however, those decisions keep me well-grounded. I am always finding new things I need to limit or new things I want to add. As long as they don't have sugar or gluten they can be a part of my plan.

IT'S NO PIECE OF CAKE

I am well aware that some do not want to make certain foods off limits. I also know that many can eat just a little bit of sugar. I have learned I can eat maybe 1 gram of added sugar if it is raw maple syrup or honey. I try not to eat more than 5 grams of added sugar a day and no processed sugar.

I use bananas if I want something I bake to have a sweet flavor. One cup of mashed bananas equals one cup of sugar. Bananas also can be substituted for butter and eggs. The sugar in fruit has water and fiber so it enters the bloodstream slower and is better for us than processed sugar or high fructose corn sugar.

Scripture does help us when we are trying to gauge what we will and won't eat. This verse really speaks to us as we examine what stays in our plan and what should go. "All things are lawful for me, but not all things are profitable. All things are lawful for you, but I will not be mastered by anything."[7]

If what I bake is something I can't stop eating that means it has the ability to master me, so I give it up. I do that because it is not profitable for me to eat something that has the ability to make me super morbidly obese again. I've come too far now to let a piece of cake or a hot roll master me even if it is gluten-free and sugar-free.

Weight loss certainly isn't a piece of cake. It's not easy and cake made with sugar is definitely something to avoid.

Like any big project we are afraid to tackle, developing a forever lifestyle change plan may look difficult, but it will lead us to the promised land of weight loss and healthier living. We will feel so much better that with God's help we won't even realize what we've done felt impossible when we began.

> Weight loss isn't easy and cake made with sugar is definitely something to avoid.

This exercise will take some time, but it will reap great benefits. Following the suggestions in this chapter and the following chapter changed my life. They will change the lives of those who are willing to develop their own forever lifestyle change plans, commit to them, and follow them with God's help.

The questions on the next page will lead you to form your own forever lifestyle change plans. It's important to spend time on this. It's not something to breeze through. This is another major key on your journey to transformation.

We all have to eat, but we don't have to eat the things that are leading us to an early death. Instead, we want to consume the foods that fuel our bodies and give us life.

QUESTIONS

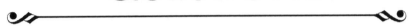

1. What things have I allowed to master me? How will this impact my forever lifestyle change plan?

2. What diets have you been on? List as many as you can remember. What about each diet worked and why did it work?

Diet	What Worked?	Why Did It Work?
1.		
2.		
3.		
4.		
5.		

3. What didn't work about the diet and why didn't it work?

Diet	What Didn't Work?	Why?
1.		
2.		
3.		
4.		
5.		

4. What might have made each diet work better? For example, was there a situation or a reason you went off the diet? Why did you gain the weight back? Was it too restrictive? Did you get bored?

5. What about your current eating plan is working? What is not working about your current plan?

6. Looking at what worked and what didn't work about all the diets you have been on as well as the way you are currently eating, what should your forever lifestyle plan include? What kind of plan will help you live a vibrant, healthy, God-centered life? Are there any things it should not include?

7. Ask God, "What do You think about this plan? Are there any adjustments I need to make? Do You have a specific plan I should be following?" Summarize what He showed you.

8. Make any adjustments in the plan and then state your forever lifestyle change plan here as succinctly as you can.

9. What is the first step you will take towards implementing this plan?

(ENDNOTES)

1. John 14:26 NIV
2. 2 Corinthians 12:9a AMP
3. 2 Corinthians 12:9b AMP
4. 2 Corinthians 12:10 AMP
5. 2 Corinthians 5:7 AMP
6. John 10:27 NIV
7. 1 Corinthians 6:12 NASB

CHAPTER 8

BUILDING TOWARDS LASTING CHANGE

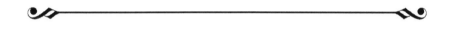

Accepting I had an issue with food, trusting God to lead me, surrendering that issue to Him, and developing my forever lifestyle change plan was difficult. As a Watchful Learner, the next step seemed like a huge leap of faith. To jump into transformation instead of going back to my own quick fix and failure, I had to allow God to build my transformation by showing me how to progressively change.

All my life I had wanted to lose weight and make it happen right now. When I got to the place where I was completely disgusted with myself for having no willpower, the only thing I knew to try was to go on another diet.

Although what we eat is a huge part of this journey, there is yet another thing we have to learn in order to implement our forever lifestyle change plan. We have to learn the discipline of how to allow God to help us change our habits. Without this piece we will continually be caught in the yo-yo dieting cycle of losing and regaining what we lost plus more.

The word diet needs to be erased from our vocabularies. We are not on a diet. We are on a forever lifestyle change journey, which will last until the day we are called home. There will never be a time when we say we've fully arrived.

We will never be perfect, but we can be growing towards spiritual maturity both in mind and character, actively integrating godly values into our daily lives.[1]

In order to do that, we have to change the habits that got us into this mess in the first place. A habit is simply a routine or a shortcut our brains use to conserve energy. We are creatures of habit. Our brains don't know a good habit from a bad. They only know there are certain things we do every day the same way at about the same time.

> A habit is simply a routine or shortcut our brains use to conserve energy.

Every morning I get up, take my morning vitamins and minerals and brush my teeth. I'm so glad I have those vitamins put into my weekly planner because some mornings I don't even remember taking them. I have to check and make sure because it's something I do without thinking. It's a habit I've built over years of doing the same thing at the same time every day.

It's also similar to going somewhere every morning at a certain time like to our work place. We get in the car and it's like our car knows exactly where to go. We just put our minds on autopilot and by habit we end up at the right place.

Our brains read our habits. They have shortcuts stored that tell us when to leave home for work and how to get there. These don't require anything more than accessing that routine for that time. It takes less energy for our brains to do that than to rethink how we are going to get to work. Then our brains are free to allow us to run through the presentation we have to do that morning and without having to think about the mundane task of getting to work.

What's really crazy is now my phone also knows this. Every weekday I go to our community pool for exercise. When I get in the car, my phone tells me how many minutes it is to get there and whether traffic is light or heavy. I didn't tell it where I was going. It didn't read my mind, but the GPS has recorded and remembers what I do. If a computer we hold in our hands can do that think what our brains can do.

GOOD AND BAD HABITS

A year or so ago my husband and I were gone for almost two weeks traveling for speaking engagements. When we got home the next morning I got up to go to exercise and my phone told me again how many minutes to the pool and what the traffic was like.

Our brains do this same thing. They remember our habits even if we've ditched them for a time period. If we try to stop a habit, but haven't put another habit in its place our phones or our brains will again suggest the habit we are trying to stop.

My phone doesn't know if the pool is a good place for me to go or not. I could be going to get donuts every morning and it would still remind me because I would have programmed it by showing it what I was doing. If I had done that one thing enough it would remind me to do it again.

To make my phone change, I would have to be in my hometown, leave from my house at that same time, and go somewhere else. When I had consistently done that for a time then my phone would automatically suggest the new route.

This is basically how we change our habits. We stop an old habit that is bad for us and start a new better habit in its place. Our brains are obviously a lot more sophisticated than a computer. We can stop a bad habit and start a good one in its place and our brains will recognize the new consistent habit if the same reward system is activated.

> We can stop a bad habit and start a good one in its place. Our brains will recognize the new consistent habit if the same reward system is activated.

For instance, if we are frustrated and we eat to comfort ourselves we can change that habit. If when we are frustrated instead of eating we do something else that will comfort us and we do that often enough, our brains will present that activity to us as the preferred option for comfort.

It could be something like listening to soothing music, journaling our thoughts, or engaging in a hobby. The key is asking God to help us be consistent with that long enough for the habit to change. Then our brains will stop tempting us with food when we need comfort and instead entice us to play soothing music.

Most psychologists use the magic number of 21 days as the time for unwanted habits to change when replaced with good ones. This is not a magic number, but the key is choosing the new habit over the old consistently for a long enough time that our brains recognize that as the preferred habit. To our brains it's about consistency, not good versus bad.

HABIT HIGHWAYS

Habits travel on a kind of nerve highway in our brains. The simple explanation is that in order to stop any habit, we must put a good habit in its place. The good habit can be anything. It doesn't have to be stopping sugar and starting to eat kale in its place. If I did that my first habit change would have failed miserably.

I call this process stop-start because I am stopping a negative habit I no longer want in my life and replacing it with a positive one. My first stop-start was to stop eating candy and to start exercising three times a week in the water for at least 30 minutes. It doesn't matter that I couldn't exercise in the water every time I wanted to eat candy. It worked for me because both were things I wanted to do. They made sense to me.

Candy had become a trigger food. It was small and easy for me to eat, so I could hide the bag in my bedroom and keep eating and eating without anyone knowing. My goal was to eventually give up all sugar, but this was early in my journey. I had surrendered sugar to God, but I still had a desire for it. I knew giving it up cold turkey would just result in me running back to it like a long lost, though evil, lover.

I was done with that, but my body still felt like it was one big blob of sugar. It was in everything I ate. To do this right I knew giving sugar up completely would just fail again like it had done when I had stopped it for limited timeframes to go on various diets. This time I was determined to do it right. I was determined to make lasting habit changes. I had to start slow and creep up on myself.

My mentor said to make our stop-starts something with a little challenge, but something we felt we could do relying on God for help. He wanted us to experience at least a small success. Small successes are great motivators. The more we have, the more we want. They keep us on the journey.

We also needed to tell our brains what we were doing. That's why we said our stop-start out loud to ourselves at home and then to our group. Our brains help us remember much better if they see it written and hear it spoken. We remember our decision better if we tell a group or at least one other person. This helps us solidify our stop-starts as firm commitments to God, others, and ourselves.

SMART GOALS

For my brain to help me understand what I wanted to do and not do, my stop-start had to be a SMART goal: Specific, Measurable, Attainable, Realistic and Timely.

Candy was all of those. It was specific. I knew exactly what it was. It was measurable because I told myself no candy, not even candies with artificial sweeteners because those simply mimic sugar and make me want sugar even more.

It was attainable because to me candy was very childish. I knew exactly why I ate it. My mother used to hide caramels in the cabinet and wouldn't let me have them. They were hers and she told me when I got to be an adult I could buy my own and eat all I wanted. I had done exactly that. Never let it be said that I didn't do what my mother told me to do!

It was realistic because I could picture the bag of candy I had in my bedroom right at that moment. The goal of giving it up was both realistic and attainable because my plan was to give the bag I had to my son the minute I got home. I'd tell him to hide it and not give me any even if I begged. I knew he was one who might eat one piece once a month. He was not a sugar addict like I was.

I was determined to make lasting habit changes. I had to start slow and creep up on myself.

I also knew because I was making the commitment to not purchase candy again, I would stick to it. Since that day all those years ago, I have stuck to that commitment.

My mentor also worked with me to make my start a SMART goal. He asked where I would exercise, when, for how long, what would constitute exercise, and how would I make sure I remembered to go.

The last was probably the most important tip he gave me. It helped me understand I had to make an appointment with myself and keep it like I would a doctor's appointment. I had to put myself first and keep the agreement I had made with myself, God, and the others who were witnessing my commitment.

For this to work, I learned I had to put firm boundaries around the stop and not think about it. It's like me telling someone not to think about a pink elephant. The more I tell them not to do that, the more they will think about that pretty pink elephant.

The same is true with sugar or anything we are trying to cut out. If we keep telling ourselves we can't eat sugar, then we are focused on the sugar. We won't focus on the great thing we want to start. Because our brains are full of the word sugar that's what we will want. That's what we have preprogrammed our brains to want as well.

When I thought of candy I pictured it with an electric fence around it. I diverted my mind to thoughts of how refreshing it would be to get back in the water that day or the next.

Candy was a no, but exercise became a deep-seated desire. After awhile I began to understand that in the past when I had been at home eating candy, it was because I was tired and wanted energy. Candy gave quick energy, but that faded as fast as it came and made me want more to get that same feeling again.

Candy was a no, but exercise became a deep-seated desire.

That cycle made me fatter, more tired, and grouchier as I endured the ups and downs of the sugar craving cycles. Exercise gave me good, lasting energy and elevated my low beta-endorphins, which made me feel awesome all day.

When I was sitting in my room eating candy, watching television or reading, I was bored and was not interacting with others. When I went to the pool I wasn't bored and I was with others. It has become a time of the day I look forward to and don't miss if at all possible.

The start has to be the focus for this to work properly. We all want to eat better, but we must agree with ourselves that the stop is a done deal and focus on the start. We need to do that by asking God for His strength and power to help us stick to our commitment.

We need to ask Him to remind us if we are going off track. Then we have to be committed to listening to His reminders and following through with His prompting. God will remind us and give us a way out of temptations[2] that seek to divert us from our stop-starts.

> A stop without a start is just another diet. It won't bring lasting change.

The problem is that many times we don't want to take that way out. The important thing here is to be aware of what God is saying.

His reminder to me is always to ask me a question to help me remember my commitment. I hear His still, small voice whisper to me, "What are you doing?" Those words then focus my brain on my overall want and I put the cookie down.

We have to understand that a stop, such as I am going to stop eating sugar, is just another diet unless we have a firm and consistent start. So many times, we focus on the stop because that seems to be the culprit.

If we over-emphasize this, we will fail. If we continually tell ourselves, no sugar, no sugar, no sugar, our brains only hear sugar, sugar, sugar. The no is silent. This is why we so often fail with a restrictive diet. A stop without a start is just another diet. It won't activate lasting change, just like a diet won't change us either.

DISMANTLE THE STOP

We try to silence the bad habit and think it will go away on its own if we try to stop thinking about it. Part of stop-start is seeing the bad habit for what it is—something that is trying to take us out of the game of life.

Eating too much sugar, starchy foods, breads, pastas, overeating any foods, binge eating, gorging, overstuffing ourselves, and engaging in what fills our fleshly desires is sin. God wants us to be done with it.

> Overeating any foods, overstuffing ourselves, eating what fills our fleshy desires ... is sin. God wants us to be done with it.

Laying it down completely has to begin with seeing it for what it is. It is a wolf in sheep's clothing. It is no longer sweet and innocent. It is a killer, plain and simple. With whatever stop we have decided on, it is necessary spend some time dismantling what we see as good about it.

Writing how this affects us is extremely helpful. Write the stop in the middle of a page of paper. It doesn't have to be food, but it could be. It could also be to stop sitting on the couch all evening, stop watching three hours television, stop being lazy by not doing laundry, stop drinking diet soda, stop going through fast food, stop eating snacks five times a day. or any other bad habit that is keeping us from being healthy.

Then we start brainstorming ways the stop has negatively affected our lives and will continue to affect us if we continue engaging it in. It can include ways engaging in this activity has caused us harm or gotten us in the shape we are in now. Write these around the stop on the page.

See the bad habit as something evil that has invaded our lives. Deconstruct it by grabbing it and seeing all the ways it has caused destruction.

We must make our brains understand the ways this habit has not been helpful to us. It is something that has captured us and is slowly taking us away from what God really wants for our lives.

BUILD THE START

In order to construct the start that we want to begin in place of the stop, think about the positive benefits of starting that new behavior. Write the start in the middle of another page and then begin to brainstorm about the great benefits that will happen when the start becomes an engrained habit. Write these around the start.

The more things we list about the positive benefits, the better. Then think of a scripture, a portion of scripture, or positive affirmation that relates to the start. Write that on another page.

> When God fulfills your longings, sweetness fills your soul.

Repeat the affirmation several times a day. Here's one of my favorite affirmations to go with stopping eating candy. "When God fulfills your longings, sweetness fills your soul."[3] One of my longings is to be healthy. I know I can't get there without intentional exercise, so this relates really well to my first stop-start.

We must be careful and not try to stop and start every single thing at once. Being overwhelmed will put us right back where we began. Start with just one stop-start. Have success with that. Small successes are great motivators.

Get that down as a consistent habit. Don't go too fast with this or it will not become incorporated firmly into your life. Work on both dismantling the stop and building the start for at least 21 days.

Once that stop-start becomes consistent, start adding other stop-starts or take that one up a notch. When I began working on my first stop-start, which was giving up candy and starting exercise, I started noticing I was going to cookies, brownies, and cakes more.

Since my main objective was to eventually give up all sugar, I began cutting those things out one at a time and adding additional exercise time. This was only 21 days after beginning my first stop-start, but because I was basically enlarging that stop-start when I had victory with stopping candy and starting exercise, it worked.

> Start with one stop-start. Small successes are great motivators.

By about six months from when I started, I had cut out processed sugar and was able to make that a firm stop. The start I added was to begin eating as much fruit as I wanted, although I limited bananas. I mainly ate strawberries or other berries in a protein shake in the mornings or in salads in the evenings. This helped eliminate my desire for sugar and gave me a fall back of a fresh fruit salad as a dessert. I still love this as my dessert.

Each stop-start has helped me look at life in a different way. No longer am I on a diet. I am looking at my life and asking God what are the bad habits I have? What are the good habits I need to start? Which one is the most important for me to work on now? How can I break it down, so I can be successful?

MAKE IT A DOABLE CHALLENGE

It's so much better to set a small, doable goal. Once we see that it is no longer challenging, start adding in other things. I did this with giving up candy first, then cookies, brownies, cakes, and sweet breads. Then, my next start was reading labels on foods to look for sugar content. What an eye opener that was!

Our tendency is to take on too much at once. This will not establish the habit firmly in our lives. We need to have patience with where we are and make sure we are establishing lasting changes that will stand through difficulties and various seasons of life.

Other stops I added were progressive ones. I stopped eating white flour, then brown flour, and then all gluten. If I saw specific foods were pulling me, I stopped those. I also adjusted bedtime by stopping work earlier, so I could get to bed earlier.

Other starts I added were learning to eat salad, learning to cook gluten-free, memorizing scripture, having solitude and silence with God each day, journaling, and reading the Bible for inspiration instead of just for study.

Also other starts were being more present with those I love, practicing being attentive to what people are saying, and intentionally neglecting things of lesser importance when I have a large project, such as a book to finish.

STOP-START IN SCRIPTURE

Stop-start is very biblical. It's all throughout the Bible. When we begin looking for it we will see the scriptures in a whole different way. There are many examples, but Romans 12:2, the well-known transformation scripture is the best.

"Do not be conformed to this world, any longer with its superficial values and customs, but be transformed and progressively changed, as you mature spiritually, by the renewing of your mind, focusing on godly values and ethical attitudes, so that you may prove for yourselves what the will of God is, that which is good and acceptable and perfect in His plan and purpose for you."[4]

We have to show our minds that we've changed our focus.

Hear the stop-start in there? Stop being conformed to the world. Start being progressively changed. Stop focusing on things that don't matter. Start renewing your mind.

Stop-start is a tool to help us reprogram our minds to help us on our healthy lifestyles. We had ourselves all set-up to run our lifestyle of who-cares-what-that-food-does-to-me-I'm-going-eat-it-anyway. We have to show our minds that we've changed our focus. We can't just tell them. We have to show them by our actions and choices. Then they will be our greatest assets.

God is all about this reprogramming project. He will help us renew our minds and change our habits if we allow Him to. We just need to ask Him to show us what needs to change in our lives so we can begin this journey to transformation.

QUESTIONS

1. What bad habits do you want to stop? List them.

1.

2.

3.

4.

5.

6.

7.

8.

9.

10.

2. What good habits do you want to start? List them.

1.

2.

3.

4.

5.

6.

7.

8.

9.

10.

3. From your list, choose a doable, but challenging, habit you want to stop. Choose a doable, but challenging, habit you want to start. Make this your first stop-start. State it with as much specificity as you can. State it so your brain knows exactly what you are intending to do and won't talk you out of it.

I will stop _____

and I will start _____

4. Run both your stop and your start through the SMART goal test. State how each is specific, measurable, attainable, realistic and timely.

5. Do the "Dismantle Your Stop "activity from this chapter. Write the stop in the center of the page and around it place words and phrases about how this has harmed you.

6. Do the "Build Your Start" activity from this chapter. Write the start in the center of the page and around it place words and phrases about how this will help you.

7. Choose a positive affirmation to repeat several times a day for 21 days. This could be a scripture or saying that reminds you of why you are doing the stop-start.

Write this in your phone, in your computer, on your refrigerator, on your mirror, or anywhere you will see it many times a day so it reminds you of the reason you are doing your stop-start. Most importantly, say it out loud.

You can download my free list of 77 Affirmations from my website to get you started.

Go to https://TeresaShieldsParker.com/77Affirmations/

(ENDNOTES)

1. Matthew 5:48 AMP
2. 1 Corinthians 10:13 NIV
3. Proverbs 13:19 TPT
4. Romans 12:2 AMP

WHOLEHEARTED TRAVELER

"Search me, O God, and know my heart, test me and know my anxious thoughts. Point out anything in me that offends You and lead me along the paths of everlasting life."

Psalm 139: 23-24 NLT

CHAPTER 9

DEALING WITH EMOTIONAL ROOTS

I was on cloud nine when I walked into the denominational headquarters where I worked. I had just gone to my weekly weigh-in for the diet I was on at the time. My dreams had come true. I had met my goal. I had lost 100 pounds!

I was 24 and this was the first time in my life I had been successful at losing weight. It had been hard. It had taken every ounce of willpower I had. I had determined to stick carefully to the plan in order to get the weight off as quickly as possible. After all, Christmas was coming. I didn't want to miss out on all those treats!

Excited to share the news with my fellow co-workers, I ran to the elevator. A department director, whom I knew in name only, held the door for me as I jumped on. I dealt with many department directors in my job, but this one traveled a lot so I didn't really know him.

He was over 40, balding and staring at me. The minute the elevator doors closed he looked me up and down and said,

"You're looking really good." I should have been elated. I should have said, "Thank you," and enjoyed the ride up to my floor. Instead, I couldn't speak or move.

PARALYZING FEAR

In my mind I was 11 years old and back in the upstairs bedroom of Grandma's house, where I was alone and about to be molested by a man I had known all my life. He was a close family friend that everyone seemed to love.

He seemed to live for enticing us girls to sit on his lap and give him kisses. In exchange he'd pull silver dollars or quarters out of our ears and give them to us. He pulled silver dollars out of the boys' ears too, but they didn't have to kiss him or sit on his lap. Even at 11, I questioned his intentions when his hands "accidentally" strayed to touch parts of my body I knew were off limits.

> I felt naked and exposed, but I could not, dared not move.

I heard the door open and saw him come in my bedroom, but I tightly shut my eyes to feign sleep. Fred[1] walked over to the bed where I was lying and commanded that I open my eyes. I didn't, but that didn't stop him. He began lifting my gown, pulling down my panties, and touching me. I was paralyzed with fear.

I felt naked and exposed, but I could not, dared not move. The situation continued while "Help me, Jesus. Help Me, Jesus" was on repeat behind my tightly closed eyes.

Right before I was sure I might be completely tainted by this man, I heard the sweetest sound in the world. "Fred, time for breakfast." It was his wife calling from the bottom of the stairs outside the room we were in.

"Be right down, Sugar," he called back.

It was several minutes before I heard the door close that I dared open my eyes for fear he might still be there waiting, lurking, and trying to catch me off guard. I caught my breath for the first time in what seemed like an eternity, but even getting my breath back couldn't calm the paralyzing fear that had taken a firm hold on me.

BACK IN THE ELEVATOR

The department director was saying words, but I couldn't seem to focus on them. I did hear him say, "We'll have to get together soon, maybe over supper?" I couldn't speak, breathe. or move.

Then the elevator doors opened to my floor. Fear shot me out of the elevator like a bullet. I ran to my office, closed the door, and buried myself in work until afternoon break.

On break, I went downstairs and ate two candy bars and drank a diet soda. I hadn't had either in at least nine months. That was the day I started gaining the weight back.

Looking back, I know the department director may or may not have been coming on to me. My emotional trigger went off, though. An older man seemed interested in my body and called attention to the fact I looked good, which I felt had to relate to my losing weight.

SNAKES

That layer of fat had always been my insulation from the kind of men I described as copperheads. I never have liked snakes, but I knew enough to know there were good snakes, like black snakes that eat mice and rodents and for those reasons are good to have around. Then there were bad snakes like poisonous copperheads, which one needs to back away from carefully or, better yet, not encounter at all.

I put Fred in the copperhead category and now the department director joined him there. I knew men who were black snakes, though, like my husband, dad, uncles, and grandfather.

They would protect me, but the problem was they couldn't be with me all the time. I figured the best way to protect myself was to make myself bigger. The good guys would still love me and the bad guys would stay away.

SILENCE IS MY WORST ENEMY

This mindset came from the 11-year-old girl inside me. I didn't tell anyone about the incident with Fred. My mother had emotional issues and I didn't think she could handle that kind of news. She would blame me thinking I had done something to entice Fred. She would be on his side.

I didn't tell my dad because I was afraid he might think the same thing. He didn't want us to wear shorts. It was summer. I was wearing shorts. Maybe it was my fault?

I didn't tell Grandma because Fred's wife was her very best friend in the whole world. She and Fred lived out of state and

Grandma looked forward to them coming every year. What if Grandma, my most favorite person in the world, would choose them over me? I couldn't live without Grandma.

I had no one to tell. So, I decided I would protect myself. I would not stay at Grandma's while they were visiting. I would keep out of Fred's way as best I could when my family was at Grandma's and I would eat to my heart's content. Maybe then he and all the men and boys like him would leave me alone.

WHAT FEAR DOES

The big problem here is that I had allowed an emotional root to be established in my life. At the time, it was impossible for me to process or understand that. What began as fear, quickly morphed into shame.

As a kid I thought I was to blame for what Fred did. If I hadn't been so attractive maybe he wouldn't have molested me. After all, he was an active church member. Surely I was the one to blame in the situation.

Back to the denominational department director in the elevator, I felt that if I had not lost weight I wouldn't have garnered that kind of response from this supposedly godly man. Within me was the overwhelming desire to run back to my old friend, sugar. Sugar would comfort and protect me.

Fear skews our perspective. Fear lies to us. Fear puts a wall between us and others. Fear seeks to render us useless to move on towards the destiny God has for us.

Fear and shame partner together to bring emotional pain into our lives. Emotional pain can feel very similar to physical pain. Emotional pain can be the start of physical symptoms of pain that no doctor can detect. We know it's there hiding in the shadows.

Usually we can manage to get through it until something triggers it again. Then we look for something quick and easy to relieve the pain. For me that was the comfort foods Grandma made. They included all kinds of desserts, but also hot rolls, hoecake, mashed potatoes, gravy, and delicious casseroles.

KNOWLEDGE HELPS

When I grew to be an adult, I began to understand the Fred issue had to be dealt with. Yet I still wasn't telling anyone it had happened. Even though Fred was deceased, I couldn't think about him without overwhelming fear. I saw him as a monster still lurking in my mind.

When I learned about pedophiles, it helped me shed some of the shame I felt. Fred was a pedophile. He was an adult who molests children, preferably girls around the age I had been. I probably wasn't the only one to whom he had done this.

They groom children by giving them things like treats or money. They choose the ones who won't tell on them because the children know and trust them. They use their influence to get what they want and their "charm" to make sure their secret is never discovered.

Then, I got mad at the fact he might have molested other girls. If I had told someone back when he did that to me maybe he would have gotten help and wouldn't have harmed others. My weight or body shape had nothing to do with what he wanted. It was my age and my gender, both of which I had no control over.

My adult mind understood the situation, but the 11-year-old me was still lost emotionally. As a rationally thinking adult I wasn't totally in charge of my emotions. The 11-year-old me was. The little girl me was still afraid and ashamed and needed the adult me to take charge and deal with the situation.

Armed with the fact that this man was in my mother's life when she was 11 and therefore could have molested her, I decided to tell my mother what happened to me. Maybe this was an emotional root festering in her for most of her life. Maybe it was the reason for the emotional illness she had dealt with for so many years.

> My adult mind understood the situation was no longer a threat, but the 11-year-old me was still lost emotionally.

When I told her, her green eyes flashed. Her voice was elevated and curt. "That never happened, and I don't ever want to hear you talk about it again."

"Mom, it did happen," I said softly.

"No, it didn't, and you are never to say anything like that again to me."

"Did he ever do anything to you?" I asked carefully.

"This is my house and you are not to speak about this again. Do you hear?" She walked out of the room and slammed the door on the subject.

That conversation reinforced my shame and increased my fear of being rejected by my family. I did tell a few select family members, but beyond that I kept to myself what seemed to be a shameful family secret that no one was supposed to find out about. The problem was that I was still living in the midst of that secret.

I shoved it down to the cellar of my life and threw food at it to keep it quiet. There it remained, growing bigger and bigger.

FORGIVENESS

"Unforgiveness is like drinking poison and hoping the other person will die." The first time I heard Joyce Meyer, now a noted Bible teacher, say those words was at one of her first conferences in St. Louis. She had not reached the recognition level she has today.

She was telling her story about being repeatedly raped by her father. As I listened it struck me that her story was 1,000 times worse than what I experienced. She talked about the fear she had of her father and how when she had forgiven him, God had set her free from both fear and shame.

As Joyce shared, I was transported to that time and space so many years ago. I pictured Fred looming over me like a huge towering hulk of a monster. I was a tiny speck. The fear was tangible.

I listened intensely as she explained that forgiveness is a process. We should make a statement to God that says, "I choose to forgive this person for what they have done to me." We hand them over to God and leave them there. If the situation comes back to our minds we do it over again. If we are diligent to do this each time the situation comes back into our thoughts, we will think of it less and less. One day we will realize the hurt is gone.

When she asked for those who had someone to forgive to stand, I stood and prayed with her. The simple prayer I prayed was, "Father God, I choose to forgive Fred for molesting me and scaring me."

All of a sudden, the monster in my mind became a shriveled up little old man. I laughed as I thought about him. I shook my head and said, "Why have I been scared of this?" I was set free from the fear of men I didn't know in an instant.

However, I still did not choose to follow the lifestyle change plan God had given me back in 1977. I had a cognitive understanding. I faced the issue emotionally. Why couldn't I go forward on my journey towards living healthy? Why couldn't I lose weight?

DEEPER CONNECTION

Sometimes God will take us back to the first time we have felt a fear and other times, He takes us back to a later incident that we have to get through first. That is what happened with this issue. Fred was a later issue that I had to address because that fear was intense. However, my inability to shed the pounds that made up my protective layer of fat was a much earlier issue that was deeply buried.

On a random day when I was exercising by jogging in our community pool, I sensed I didn't trust Jesus. So I asked Him if I trusted Him and I got no response. For me, this usually means there is wall between us. I asked Jesus to show me the wall. He did and we were able to remove it, which in and of itself was not easy.[2]

I sensed we had done an important work, but I knew I was still not ready to trust Jesus to completely lead me. Not being able to trust a member of the Godhead usually means I have a root of fear, but I had no sense of why it was there. It seemed really buried. I've learned to simply leave it with God and He will reveal it in His time.

I continued to exercise and after some time, Jesus dropped a memory into my mind. It was a time Adam,[3] a seven-year-old boy in our neighborhood, misled me by asking me to play doctor and nurse with him in his fort. I was six years old.

> Not being able to trust someone usually means I have a root of fear.

I thought that meant playing with the nurse kit I got for Christmas. I was happy to be included, but I had no idea I was not to be the nurse. I was the patient, who was thoroughly "examined" by the "doctor."

Later when I was 16, Adam came back for a visit and asked me to go out for a soda to talk and maybe see a movie. Mom said that was OK as long as we didn't go to the drive-in movie. Adam agreed with a "Yes, Ma'am."

Like an inexperienced teenager, I trusted Adam would keep his promise. Instead, he again misled me by going directly to the drive-in movie theater. He didn't even know what movie was playing. He had other things on his mind.

I was barely able to halt his efforts and convince him take me home because he promised not to take me to the drive-in and if we got back too late, both Dad and Mom would know. Adam was mad, which suited me just fine. He had been a companion, but he misled me. I had given him a second chance, but he had not changed.

I understood that I had to forgive Adam for using and manipulating me, but I wasn't sure how that was going to connect to my lack of trust in Jesus. I started by saying, "Jesus, I choose to forgive Adam for misleading me about his intentions, not once but twice. I choose to forgive him for making me believe he liked me as a person and wanted my company when what he really wanted was a thrill. I forgive him for making me feel dirty and sinful. I forgive him for making me afraid of trusting men."

> It was residing in me as an emotional root until I finally confronted it and allowed Jesus to help me pull it out.

Jesus is my companion, the one who walks and talks with me, the member of the Godhead who understands my human condition. When childhood companions do something that hurts me in some way, I may begin to transfer that same kind of feeling to Jesus. As an adult I know it isn't true, but as a child I never processed it, so it was residing in me as an emotional root until I finally confronted it and allowed Jesus to help me pull it out.

I continued my prayer. "I renounce the lie that You, Jesus, will mislead me. You will take me places I don't want to go. You will place me in situations where I cannot make right choices. I renounce the lie You say You want to get to know me, but it's only to get me on Your side to use me for Your benefit. You just want me to be Your slave. I renounce the lie that in order to get Your attention, I have to do things I don't want to do. I renounce the lie I can never trust You."

I always know when I have gotten to the root of an issue. None of those lies had ever surfaced in my conscious mind, but I saw exactly how they were governing my mistrust. I was anxious to know the answer to the next question. "Jesus, what is Your truth?"

I sensed Him revealing many things to me, but what stood out was, "I called John the beloved disciple because He understood what I was about. I entrusted My mother to him.[4]

"I only entrust my prized possessions to those I trust. I love you, Teresa, but more than that, I trust you because I know your heart. I claimed you as my bride. You are my beloved.[5]"

HOW GOD VIEWS FORGIVENESS

It never ceases to amaze me how this process of forgiveness works to set me free from past emotional roots I didn't even know were there until God revealed them to me.

Forgiveness is rooted in God's love. He loved us so much that He forgave us. Now, we must forgive others.[6] Love is the opposite of fear. "There is no room in love for fear. Well-formed love banishes fear."[7] Love formed as forgiveness does away with fear. Love roots fear out and destroys it.

In the model prayer Jesus asks us to pray, "Forgive us the wrongs we have done as we ourselves release forgiveness to those who have wronged us.[8] For if you withhold forgiveness from others, your Father withholds forgiveness from you.[9]"

Forgiveness is one of the ultimate expressions of God's love. It is a tool He gives us to set us free. God asks us to forgive others because He knows it is the only thing that enables us to not live under emotional bondage of what another person has done to us.

Forgiveness leads to our freedom. The department director was not the problem. Fred really wasn't the root problem. Adam was. Though I did go through forgiveness for both of them, it really was the situation with Adam that held the biggest key for me.

RENOUNCING LIES

To get there I had to forgive Him, renounce the lie that Jesus would treat me that way and ask Him, "What is Your truth?" Hearing, seeing or sensing God's truth is where the real emotional freedom comes. On some cognitive adult level, we know what the truth is, but when we allow God to tell us His truth it makes all the difference in the world. It becomes a personal experience no one can take from us.

Many times, when I go through this process I picture God, sitting on the edge of His throne leaning in just waiting for me to ask Him the one question that will bring me freedom. "What is Your truth?"

It is not enough to rationally know or understand the words that are factual, we have to experience that truth. It's when we experience His truth that we are set free.[10] It is a personal experience for us when we know God has spoken directly to us, dropped a truth in our heart, shown us a picture, or we have sensed His presence. No one can take that from us.

Confronting the emotional roots that have kept us in bondage for years helps us resolve why we have not been able to go forward. It is because in some way, we feel God will treat us the same way as other humans who have mistreated us.

Mothers, fathers, siblings, companions all may play a part in the emotional roots we are afraid to face. I totally get it. I understand why we are afraid.

> I didn't want to face the Fred monster or the Adam Manipulator, but when I did it in a safe environment I was set free.

Many I work with have felt if they ignore the hurts of their past they will go away. It rarely does. If we feel trapped in fear and emotional bondages, we need to reach out to a Christian coach who has been there or a counselor who understands what we are feeling.

I didn't want to face the Fred monster or the Adam Manipulator, but when I did it in a safe environment I was set free. Establishing a safe environment to help others find their freedom from fear and emotional bondages is the reason I do one-on-one coaching..

Hearing what God says or seeing what He shows us in a time of prayer and reflection helps release us from emotional bondages. We finally are able to experience who God really is in our lives. Most of those I'm able to help tell me afterwards they feel free, much lighter or like they are floating. I love being a part of these sessions.

I no longer eat to protect myself from men who might harm me. I love meeting and interacting with new people, even men. I don't automatically assume every man is a copperhead snake.

I've been in situations where I could have assumed a man I didn't know was having bad intentions toward me, however in every situation they were just being friendly. For me to get to the point where I can see friendly as a good thing is a huge breakthrough.

I know the difference between healthy caution and a spirit of fear. God gives us awareness and has built in to us the adrenalin we need to get us out of situations which will bring us harm. He did not, however, give us a spirit of fear. He gave us love, power, and a sound mind.[11]

I have God's strength and power in any given situation combined with a sound mind to think through what is really happening. When I mix in the love of God, I am able to live my life without fear directing what I put in my mouth.

I no longer hide behind a mound of weight to protect myself or keep others away lest they find out some deep, dark secrets. I am no longer afraid and think every man is somehow out to harm me. Living in fear is no way to live.

> I have God's strength and power in any given situation combined with a sound mind to think through what is really happening. When I mix in the love of God, I am able to live my life without fear

I love being the person God designed me to be. I love being His Bride, His Beloved, one He can trust. If He can trust me, I surely can trust Him.

QUESTIONS

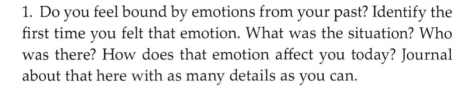

1. Do you feel bound by emotions from your past? Identify the first time you felt that emotion. What was the situation? Who was there? How does that emotion affect you today? Journal about that here with as many details as you can.

2. The next step is forgiveness. Write a list of everything you need to forgive the person for that you just wrote about. This should include specific ways they made you feel or specific things they did. Once you have listed these things say out loud, "I choose to forgive _____ for _____" (all the things you just listed).

3. Say out loud, "I renounce the lie that God, Jesus or Holy Spirit will treat me the way the person treated me whom I just forgave." Say the specific things you listed in question 2 and just forgave that person for. These are lies you are renouncing about God.

4. Say out loud, "God, Jesus or Holy Spirit, what is Your truth?" Write down the first thing you see, hear or feel. Remember you just asked the God of the universe a question. He will answer you. If you see, hear or feel something you don't understand, ask Him what it means. This is a conversation between you and God. If you need clarity at any time, ask.[12]

5. What did God show you through this exercise? Be sure to write down what He gave you as truth. Journal about this time. Repeat this process when new emotions come to the forefront.

(ENDNOTES)

1. Not his name.

2. See chapter 15 of Teresa's book, *Sweet Freedom: Losing Weight and Keeping It Off with God's Help*, https://www.amazon.com/Sweet-Freedom-Losing-Weight-Keeping/dp/0991001257

3. Not his name.

4. John 19:27 NLT

5. Deuteronomy 33:12 NIV, Song of Songs 6:3 NIV

6. Ephesians 4:32 NLT, Colossians 3:13 NLT

7. 1 John 4:18 MSG

8. Matthew 6:12 TPT

9. Matthew 6:15 TPT

10. John 8:32 MSG

11. 2 Timothy 7-8 NKJV

12. For more information about healing emotional roots, see Teresa's books, *Sweet Freedom Study Guide*, https://www.amazon.com/Sweet-Freedom-Study-Guide-Keeping/dp/0991001273/ or of *Sweet Freedom: Losing Weight and Keeping It Off with God's Help*, https://www.amazon.com/Sweet-Freedom-Losing-Weight-Keeping/dp/0991001257

OVERCOMING DISCOURAGEMENT

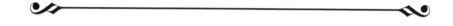

When we get the stage of Wholehearted Traveler on it can seem like everything begins to happen to take us off course. We may say, like I have many times, "Hey God, I went on this journey to have a better life not be overwhelmed by my life."

At times my discouragement has been so huge that it felt like I had lost any and all courage to face the difficulties life had thrown my way. One truth I have learned to hold onto, though, is that no matter what is happening in my life or the lives of those I love, God is right there with me slogging through the pain.

If we allow difficulties to overwhelm us, we have succumbed to one of the enemy's biggest ways to try to throw us off course. If he can pull the courage out of us, then fear can take over. When we open the door to fear nothing we do will change that as long as we are fully living in the land of panic and anxiety.

To be discouraged means to have a loss of confidence or enthusiasm about life. It's as if we have been cut off from the courage to keep going and face everyday life. We don't want to risk again. We don't want to try to lose weight again. It would dishearten us if it didn't work. It would frustrate and dismay us.

To keep ourselves anywhere near sane we decide to give up trying to change. Giving up seems easier than trying and failing again. We just can't take another defeat. To avoid that we live in the land of denial and fantasy that says everything is fine with me.

We live in the land of denial and fantasy that says everything is fine with me.

I did this time and again throughout my life. I loved losing weight. I looked forward to achieving a great goal, like losing 100 pounds. Reaching any goal was always a high. I loved being able to say, "I did it! Look at me go!"

Unfortunately, I also looked forward to rewarding myself with one of my favorite desserts. When I'd do that, it would send me back on the quest to eat whatever I wanted, whenever I wanted. Then it wouldn't take long to gain back the weight I'd lost plus more.

I know beyond a shadow of a doubt that the body desires to inflate those fat cells again as quick as it can. I had programmed my body to welcome that weight plus more to come back and settle in.

As soon as I started back eating unhealthy food, I'd forget what healthy living felt and tasted like. I'd forget that when I was eating healthy, I felt better physically. I looked better. My brain was clearer. My energy level was up.

When I returned to sugar, my drug of choice, everything would go downhill. I didn't know what was happening because my brain cells were filled with sugar again. At some point in time, I would be awakened from a deep comfortable sleep to the nightmare of realizing I had gained 100 pounds back plus more. That's when the major discouragement would hit me again.

ENCOURAGEMENT

Encouragement never kicked in after I lost weight because I didn't give it time. When someone would try to give me a compliment, it just seemed to make me want to eat more.

It felt like an insult robed in praise. I felt they were really saying, "Glad you lost weight because you were really fat." While that was true, it still discouraged me. They were making a positive observation, but I felt like they didn't deserve to make that statement because they hadn't walked a mile in my shoes.

Weight loss didn't happen for me until a real encourager came along. This wasn't a person who sat on the outside observing what was happening and telling me what I should do and not do.

This was someone who gave me support and didn't treat me like I was a needy fat blob. He became a mentor to me because he not only answered my questions when I asked them, but he instilled confidence in me by telling me how these suggestions had worked in his own life.

That gave me hope that the tools would work for me. For the first time someone boosted my morale and inspired me to work on myself because I am worth it. Loving and taking care of myself is my first assignment from God so that I can fulfill the destiny He has for me.

> In this one area, I felt the absence of God's Spirit. It felt like He was working in every other area of my life, but not this one.

The best thing my mentor did was always point me to God. He let me know if I would allow God to help me, the way to fulfilling my destiny would be made clear.

When I would gain back the weight I had lost I became dispirited, which means the same thing as being disheartened or losing hope. I was a Christian, but in this one area I felt the absence of God's Spirit. It felt like He was working in every other area of my life, but not this one.

It unnerved me to think that the Holy Spirit would be absent in any area of my life. Of course, He wasn't. It was just that sugar, breads, desserts, and starchy foods had filled my need for Him. He was my comforter, but I was interested in using something more tangible like food to provide a false comfort.

I had no idea how to taste and see that the Lord is good.[1] That made absolutely no sense to me. I didn't understand that what I had done was replace the Holy Spirit with my own desires. When I am led by my wants and desires I will always go contrary to God's Spirit.

When I try to circumvent what the Holy Spirit is telling me it will always lead me into discouragement. One way I step into this sense of disappointment with who I am is to want what I want, thus going against what God wants for me.

This is very similar to how it feels when life throws us curve balls. Something happens out of the blue like a disease, accident, job loss, death, or divorce. These are things we can't control. We want to fix them, but we can't.

Then discouragement sets in and we are dispirited. We get down on ourselves and dig a pit we can't seem to climb out of. We just know there is a black cloud of doom, despair and agony that is following us around. No matter how hard we try we cannot see the silver lining in that cloud.

DAVID'S DISCOURAGEMENT

David was discouraged many times. Yet God said, "I have found David, son of Jesse, a man after my own heart."[2] David handled discouragement by admitting it head-on to God.

He said, "As the deer longs for streams of water, so I long for you, O God. I thirst for God, the living God. When can I go and stand before him? Day and night, I have only tears for food, while my enemies continually taunt me, saying, 'Where is this God of yours?'

"My heart is breaking as I remember how it used to be: I walked among the crowds of worshipers, leading a great procession to the house of God, singing for joy and giving thanks amid the sound of a great celebration!

"Why am I discouraged? Why is my heart so sad? I will put my hope in God! I will praise him again—my Savior and my God. Now I am deeply discouraged, but I will remember you—even from distant Mount Hermon, the source of the Jordan, from the land of Mount Mizar.

"I hear the tumult of the raging seas as your waves and surging tides sweep over me. But each day the Lord pours his unfailing love upon me, and through each night I sing his songs praying to God who gives me life.

"O God, my rock,' I cry, 'Why have you forgotten me? Why must I wander around in grief, oppressed by my enemies?' Their taunts break my bones. They scoff 'Where is this God of yours?'

"Why am I discouraged? Why is my heart so sad? I will put my hope in God! I will praise him again—my Savior and my God!'"[3]

WHAT'S GOING ON?

David wrote this at a time when he was not able to go to the sanctuary to worship God. For David, God was in that space. David was desperate for God. Sometimes it is only in our moments of despair and suffering that we desire God even more.

Discouragement and despair will garner one of two reactions towards God. We will either get mad at God or draw closer to God. In his discouragement, David wisely chose to do the latter. He was drawing closer to God, panting for God, thirsting for the living water of God. He was so distraught he wasn't even eating. He longed to worship God the way He had always known. In verse two he said, "When can I go and stand before Him?"

David remembered how it used to be when he was loved by the people, then he remembered how the crowd seemed to be against him. Even with this he acknowledged God and His unfailing love. He prayed and sang to God in the midst of what looks like a bleak time.

He was honest with God and admitted his discouragement and sadness. He still stood on the fact that his secure hope was in God as his Savior. He once again was honest about his discouragement, but he also remembered and acknowledged God.

None of us can solve our problems by worrying them to death.

When we are in the middle of heart-breaking discouragement, we must admit it to God. Hiding it will only intensify our discouragement. Healing only comes when we are truthful with God and ourselves. Denial never works to help us see things clearly.

We acknowledge where we are and know that God will bring us through this season with greater wisdom, insight, and knowledge to face our next season. We can do this because experience has taught us there is no other place to go for help in times of need, but to the one who will hold us through our discouragement.

None of us can solve our problems by worrying them to death. We have to be honest with God before we can be honest with ourselves and understand that we cannot fix our problems. Problems will lead us to a deeper understanding of who God is and how He works.

We must admit that in our own human strength our problem is beyond our ability to cope with. We have to understand that God may not fix our emotional angst right then, but because He has never failed us we will choose to trust His sovereignty.

This doesn't mean that there won't be some suffering along the way. Suffering and pain is a result of the entrance of sin into the world. It is not of God. God is sovereign. He doesn't remove the suffering but uses our difficulties to draw us closer to Him.

In the midst of discouragement, the one thing we must do is get as close to God as possible. Seek Him. Cry out to Him. Tell Him the truth of how we feel, but then lay our heads on His chest and rest in His embrace. That's the only proper position to wait on Him.

When we come close to God, then God will come close to us.[4] The first move is ours.

GOOD OUT OF BAD

God weaves our joys with sorrows, triumphs with tragedies, and successes with failures to fit into His perfect plan of bringing good into our lives because we are His lovers who have been called to fulfill His designed purpose.[5]

Being in the midst of discouragement, difficulty, sorrow, and despair, seems to be the only time we remember to be 100 percent dependent on God.

Many times we think we can control the outcome with just a quickly spoken prayer. We don't cry out to Him for our very lives and the lives of those we love. We simply take everything for granted.

Sure, we tell Him, thank You, but we don't grasp the depths of what He has done for us until we face mountains we know are certainly not removable by any act of ours.

We have to understand that the lessons we learn in the valleys will lead us to the mountaintops to worship God as the only Giver of the true abundance this life brings.

> The lessons we learn in the valleys will lead us to the mountaintops to worship God on as the only Giver of the true abundance this life brings.

It is in times of discouragement and despair that we come to the end of ourselves, admit our complete weakness, and begin to rely on His strength 100 percent.

Discouragement exposes our weak areas. When we see those we shouldn't try harder. We should seek God's strength more.

Notice that one thing David did was sing to God. He said, "Through each night I sing His songs, praying to God who gives me life."[6]

When we are in the midst of despair and need to encourage ourselves, we need to proclaim who we know God to be to us. We need to join David and sing a new song to God. We need to pray and make declarations about who God is in our lives. More than anything a song will lift our spirits as we honestly sing it to God with our whole hearts.

In the midst of discouragement, when there is no one near to encourage us, we need to encourage or strengthen ourselves in the Lord.[7]

GIVE ENCOURAGEMENT

Encourage means to give support, confidence or hope to someone. It's when we uplift, inspire, motivate, invigorate, revitalize or fire up others or ourselves. It is actually putting courage back into our lives.

The scriptures impart to us encouragement and inspiration so that we can live in hope and endure all things.[8]

Many places in the New Testament talk about our role as encouragers towards others. We are to discover creative ways to encourage others and to motivate them toward acts of compassion, doing beautiful works as expressions of love.[9] As we encourage others, we will also find that we are encouraging ourselves.

You can get glad in the same pants you got mad or sad in.

My Grandma used to tell me, "You can get glad in the same pants you got sad or mad in." She was telling me to focus on the positive instead of the negative. She told me if I was down or sad to just start telling God the things I am thankful for rather than the things I am upset about.

When I am discouraged and think God is not seeing me or doesn't know what's happening in my life, I start telling Him, "Thank You." Then I list every blessing starting with the people who are most dear to me. It immediately brings me into His presence.

When discouragement hits, it is not a time to hide from God. It is a time to draw closer. Getting alone with God in stillness and solitude away from all distractions is the first step. We

182

invite Him into our refuge and ask Him to correct any lies we have about Him or our current situation. Then we simply wait and listen for His answer.

That can come in a variety of ways, but I find when I ask God a direct question He will answer me with the first thing I hear, see, or feel. It's a matter of paying attention. God tells us, "Call to me and I will answer you and tell you great and unsearchable things you do not know."[10]

> **The best way to forgive ourselves is to simply get back on that horse and ride with God's help.**

We must also repent for anything we have done that we are discouraged about. We forgive ourselves for any way in which we have been a party to causing our own discouragement.

When we mess up we depress ourselves. We wish we hadn't done that. No one did us wrong. We did that all by ourselves. Many times, I had to forgive myself when I gained weight. This was no one else's fault. It was definitely a discouragement I brought on myself.

The best way to forgive ourselves is to simply get back on that horse and ride with God's help. He does long to help us. We ask God to forgive us for messing up. Then ask Him for a plan to set us back on course again and we ask for His strength to help us follow that plan.

We must be truthful with God about how we feel. There have been times I've said to God, "God, it really is the pits that I can't eat sugar. It stinks that I can just look at food and gain weight. Still I know You love me and have good plans for my life. Remind me of who I am and what Your desires are for me."

I've learned to repeat His promises, quote scriptures, and read the Bible out loud. I especially like to read the Psalms and highlight the verses that speak to me about who God is to me and who I am to Him. More than anything I thank Him for how He has led me in the past, what He has brought me through, and how He has been faithful to me.

I know whatever difficulty I'm going through will lead to something deeper and greater or I wouldn't be going through it. Being assured of that, I thank God for how He is leading me in the midst of my current crisis.

ENCOURAGE OURSELVES IN THE LORD

When I am discouraged it helps to intentionally encourage someone else. I might send a card or email to someone, share a meaningful scripture on Facebook, give a compliment, double my tip to a waiter or waitress, or take a gift to a neighbor or someone in need.

Another way I encourage myself is listening to great Christian music. I especially like to find a new contemporary Christian song and let it fill me with new hope and awe-struck wonder of who God really is in my life.

I can never be discouraged when I'm remembering all God's attributes. Praising Him for who He is, telling Him I can't live without Him is one of the best ways to step over the line from discouragement into encouragement.

Let us encourage ourselves in the Lord.[11]

QUESTIONS

1. When is the last time you got away with God for an extended time and really opened your heart to Him? If it's been awhile, don't overwhelm yourself. Still, set aside at least an hour to do that. If you regularly spend time with God, spend more time than usual. You can use this page to journal about what He shares with you.

2. What are you discouraged about? With gut-level honesty admit that to God.

3. Is there any way in which you have contributed to your own discouragement by not doing what you committed to doing? Ask God to forgive you for that. Ask Him to give you a new plan to go forward on your journey. Covenant with Him that you will follow what He tells you.

4. How has God led you in the past? What has He brought you through? How has He been faithful to you? What blessings has He given you? Write these down and as you do, thank Him for all He has done.

5. What is one specific thing you can do to encourage someone today? Write about what you did.

(ENDNOTES)

1. Psalm 34:8 NIV
2. Acts 13:22 NIV
3. Psalm 42:1-11 NLT
4. James 4:8 NLT
5. Romans 8:28 TPT
6. Psalm 42:8 NLT
7. 1 Samuel 30:6 NKJV
8. Romans 15:4 TPT
9. Hebrews 10:24 TPT
10. Jeremiah 33:3 NIV
11. 1 Samuel 30:6 KJV

WISE OVERCOMER

"So I am well-pleased with weaknesses, with insults, with distresses, with persecutions and with difficulties for the sake of Christ. For when I am weak in human strength then I am strong, truly able, truly powerful, truly drawing from God's strength."

2 Corinthians 12:10 AMP

A LESSON IN HUMILITY

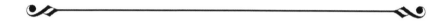

The two-story farmhouse was situated on the top of a hill overlooking 500 acres of lush pastureland fed by Hungry Mother Creek. In the back of the house was the chicken coop where Grandma gathered eggs every morning. On the top of the hill was the barn, out-buildings, tractors, wagons, and barn lot, all things us grandchildren loved to explore.

To me, my grandparent's farm was more home than my parent's house. Although the farmhouse was not fancy or pretentious in any way, it was much larger than the 800 square-foot house where my family lived about 30 miles away.

GOD AS PROVIDER

I don't know how old I was when my mom told me that my grandparents were considered to be some of the wealthier farmers in their area. During the Depression my grandfather, whom we called Papaw, was working for a wealthy horse rancher. The man bought and sold racehorses and Papaw raised and trained them. He was able to save money during that time. After the Depression the man sold him the best farmland on his ranch.

My grandparents, though, didn't act like they had a lot of money. Of course, we got beef, pork, chickens, and all the fresh produce we could pick, but I just figured that was because they were our grandparents who owned a farm. I didn't realize it was worth a lot of money.

They weren't haughty, arrogant, or prideful. They came from ordinary farm families. They considered what happened to them as being in the right place at the right time, but they also gave credit to God as their provider. That wasn't just lip service. I saw that lived out in their lives.

I can still remember listening to Papaw and Grandma praying together each night after they turned the lights out. I would either be on a pallet beside their bed or in the upstairs bedroom right above theirs with the window open. I heard them pray for me, for each family member, for their church, for their animals and crops, and for people in the community. I knew Papaw's heart most from his prayers and his actions.

GOOD DEEDS

One thing I remember about Papaw was going with him to take several dozen eggs to Bill and George every week. These were two bachelor brothers who lived less than five miles from my grandparents. One of them was bedfast. The other did the cooking. Papaw said he took them eggs, so he knew they'd have something to eat. He knew they ate the eggs because they would hand their empty cartons back to him as if gold bars he had lent to them.

Papaw would stay and talk to them while I played ...the dog outside. The inside of the house smelled too bad for me to stay for long, but it never seemed to bother Papaw. When I asked why he went every week, he said he wanted to make sure they didn't need anything because they didn't have a phone.

Even though he had money and was well known in the community, Papaw loved every person the same. He had no pride in his standing. When I think of a humble person, I think of Papaw.

PRIDE IS A WALL WE BUILD

Pride is an easy sin to fall into if one has lots of money, power, and achievements. Most of the time we relegate pride to those types of people. I can say from first-hand experience, that's not all that's involved in pride.

The biblical definition of pride is ultimate confidence in self, instead of God. Other words to describe pride include stubborn, willful, arrogant, and haughty. When I was super morbidly obese I never thought of myself as prideful. I was ashamed of myself, didn't like myself, and was constantly angry with myself. I did not think I was proud. However, pride was a huge wall I had built to keep others out.

I thought of myself all the time and indulged myself constantly with foods I loved. I was stubborn and willful for sure. I was in all ways prideful because I catered to my own wants at any price.

Sometimes we think if we feel poorly about ourselves, then that means we are humble. Actually, when we feel bad about ourselves and then eat to try to take care of the pain we are still self-absorbed. Anytime we are putting our selfish needs first we are in pride.

HUMILITY IS SUBMISSION TO GOD

A Wise Overcomer is one who has learned that humility is being in complete submission to God. When we submit to God and put Him and what He wants first we have laid down our selfishness and are seeking only what He desires. This is true humility. It simply means we are putting God first in every area. We are dedicated to following Him even in what we eat and how we move.

How do we obtain humility and work against pride? Why is all this important to God? James 4 has the answer. It's the first chapter of the Bible I ever memorized.

I knew I had a problem with food and I knew it was a spiritual issue, but I couldn't put my finger on the exact nature of the problem. Even after memorizing James 4 it took years for me to actually implement what this passage points out.

"What is the source of quarrels and conflicts among you? Is not the source your pleasures that wage war in your members?

"You lust and do not have; so, you commit murder. You are envious and cannot obtain; so, you fight and quarrel. You do not have because you do not ask. You ask and do not receive, because you ask with wrong motives, so that you may spend it on your pleasures.

"You adulteresses, do you not know that friendship with the world is hostility toward God? Therefore, whoever wishes to be a friend of the world makes himself an enemy of God. Or do you think that the scripture speaks to no purpose: 'He jealously desires the Spirit which He has made to dwell in us?'

"But He gives a greater grace. Therefore, it says, 'God is opposed to the proud, but gives grace to the humble.'

"Submit therefore to God. Resist the devil and he will flee from you. Draw near to God and He will draw near to you. Cleanse your hands, you sinners; and purify your hearts, you double-minded.

"Be miserable and mourn and weep; let your laughter be turned into mourning and your joy to gloom. Humble yourselves in the presence of the Lord, and He will exalt you."[1]

PERSONAL APPLICATION

Paraphrasing a passage so I see how it relates to my specific issue helps me apply the truths more directly to my point of need. I rewrote James 4 to step on my own toes and shake a little sense into myself. I did it to be better able to apply the truth from this passage to my life.

"What is the source of the double-mindedness in me that causes me to have quarrels and conflicts within myself? Isn't it the fact that I want to eat the things that bring me pleasure? Because of that I am constantly at war with myself because I know it is not healthy for me.

"I crave the foods I love and am never satisfied. I am slowly killing myself. Still I want more, so I am angry and fight with myself. I don't have because I do not ask with the right motives. I don't really want food to help me live. I want the foods I want because they bring me pleasure.

"I am like an adulteress because I am cheating on God by desiring only things that fill my own pleasure. When I crave the things of this world more than God, I become an enemy of God. The Word tells me the Holy Spirit must reign in me instead of my human spirit with its desires for the foods I crave.

"God's overflowing grace, which is the power of the Holy Spirit to meet my earthly desires and evil tendencies, is my salvation in every way. When I want what I want instead of what God wants for me, I am proud and haughty and God sets Himself against what I want. But when I am humble and submit myself fully to God, He gives me grace continually.

> When I crave the things of this world more than God, I become an enemy of God.

"Therefore, I will bow to God in every way. I will stand firm against the devil and His temptations and He will run from me. I will draw near to God and when I do, I know He will draw near to me. I will ask for forgiveness, turn from my wrong ways, and allow God to cleanse my heart. I realize I have been wavering and have had divided interests. I have not put God first. Today, I stop being wishy-washy and I put Him first.

"I repent for what I have done wrong. I am remorseful and deeply sorry. I grieve over how I have not been loyal to my God. This is the first step to humbling myself in God's sight. And although I don't do it to be exalted, I know that when I finally put God first, I cannot help but be lifted up as I step into my right standing as His child."[2]

BREAKING IT DOWN

When we break down this passage and how it applies to us, we have to look at seven themes it brings up.

1. Being double-minded is the beginning of a root of pride. For me that was wanting to eat whatever I wanted in the moment and wanting to follow God. We can't have it both ways. Even if what we want to eat in the moment is not "bad" food, if we know God is telling us not to then we need to show Him by our actions that we are choosing to follow Him.

2. We are like adulteresses when we follow our human spirits instead of God's Spirit. Our God is a jealous God. He wants us to have no other gods before Him, especially not our stomachs.[3]

3. Grace is the power of the Holy Spirit to help me. It reveals to me that I need to humble myself and submit to

> Grace is the power of the Holy Spirit to help me.

God. When I do that, I get even more grace. If I don't do that, I am in pride and God must oppose me because I am acting against Him. If I'm not with Him, I am against Him.

4. When I submit fully to God in every way only then am I a child of obedience and can stand firm against the devil.

I can say, "No devil. I am a child of obedience to my Lord and Savior Jesus Christ. I will no longer listen to you. Go away and leave me alone in Jesus' name." Then that old devil will turn tail and run!

5. When I draw near to God, He draws near to me. When the pride is gone and humility has entered I am ready to stop being a person who wavers with each choice.

> Those who humble themselves will receive the honor of being exalted.

6. Humility requires my heart-felt repentance. It's not just something I say. It's something I do and live out each day. I must understand completely what I've done.

It's not a quick, "I'm sorry." It's something that grieves me deeply to the point that I feel the pain of what I have done. It's more than words. The status of my heart changes from what I want to what God wants for me. "Humans see only what is visible to the eyes, but the Lord sees into the heart."[4]

7. Even though we don't become humble in order to be exalted, those who humble themselves will receive the honor of being exalted. It only comes, though, when being exalted is the last thing on our minds.

The humble person has gotten rid of all their selfish desires and wants. They have laid them on the altar. They don't want them anymore. They have given up all earthly motives of power, money, and pleasure. These are worthless to the humble person.

Only when we have let go of every earthly motive are we able to truly draw near to God. That's when we begin to feel His presence and hear His heartbeat. When we draw near to Him in moments of intimacy we are exalted in God's eyes.

"Those who think themselves great shall be disappointed and humbled; and those who humble themselves shall be exalted."[5] We can only begin to understand what it means to receive God's pleasure when we have humbled ourselves by repenting and turning away from things that we know do not bring God pleasure.

Humility leads to a closer relationship with God, which leads us to experience more of God's favor. When we are humble, we aren't asking for His favor. We aren't that child with her hand out. We're the child totally dependent and totally trusting in God, His provision, His protection, and His guidance.

"The high and lofty one who lives in eternity, the Holy One, says this: 'I live in the high and holy place with those whose spirits are contrite and humble. I restore the crushed spirit of the humble and revive the courage of those with repentant hearts."[6]

God answers all prayers, but when we are humble we choose to draw close to Him first in times of trouble. Because of that intimacy He will take care of us, restore us, and revive us.

> **If God wants to use us and we aren't humble already He will set up circumstances to create humility within us.**

He does this because He knows our hearts are truly humble. We no longer depend on our own strength. We depend on God. When we depend completely on Him, He lifts our spirits.

If God wants to use us and we aren't humble already He will set up circumstances to create humility within us. That's exactly what He did with me on my weight loss journey. He also did it with the children of Israel.

"The Lord your God led you all the way these 40 years in the wilderness, to humble you and test you, to know what *was* in your heart, whether you would keep His commandments or not. So, He humbled you, allowed you to hunger, and fed you with manna, which you did not know nor did your fathers know, that He might make you know that man shall not live by bread alone; but man lives by every word that proceeds from the mouth of the Lord."[7]

> God knows if we are truly thankful for the food He provides or resentful that it isn't what we want to eat.

The entire purpose of the 40-year journey through the wilderness was to humble the children of Israel and test them. Most of them didn't pass the test. Hunger was one of those tests. It took me 30 years to pass the hunger test.

The test for the children of Israel wasn't whether or not they would eat the manna. The test was whether they would be satisfied with what He gave them to eat. It was also a test to see if they grumbled and complained or not and if they followed God's instructions or not.

God knows our hearts. He knows if we are truly thankful for the food He provides or resentful that it isn't what we want. He knows what we crave and He knows what we crave isn't what He has shown us is best for us to eat in order to fuel our bodies. At times I prayed for manna so I could eat only what God wanted me to eat. If He had given me manna, though,

I would have been like the children of Israel. I would have grumbled and complained. I wouldn't have been satisfied.

We must recognize pride when it seeps in. Sometimes it happens when we are at a family dinner or out with friends at a restaurant and we want to fit in and be like everyone else. We know there are things we could choose to eat that will be death for us instead of life, but our pride won't let us say no to these things.

Humble people would not take any dessert or not order any or not look longingly at the desserts of those who did order them. Humble people follow what God shows them to do.

> Humble people take time to draw near to God. They make it a priority in their lives.

Humble people take time to draw near to God. They make it a priority in their lives. They understand this entire life journey is all about drawing near to God rather than to the dessert or the big meal we want to eat.

Humble people do not make physical pleasures, like the food they want for supper, become what they are craving and looking forward to all day. They focus on the times they get to spend in the presence of God. Their priorities are centered on how He is leading them.

Humble people understand one thing God wants is for them to prosper and be in good health physically, even as their souls prosper spiritually.[8] Taking care of ourselves physically means we are humbling ourselves to do what God wants for us. Humble people obey and follow what God shows them to do.

THE CRAVING TEST

Today our test is do we live by spiritual food or physical food? Do we crave those special times with God where He seems so close we can touch Him? Do we crave those times when it feels like He is holding us close and whispering the mysteries of the universe? Do we crave just being in the presence of the God of the universe?

> Bread alone will not satisfy, but true life is found in every word, which constantly goes forth from God's mouth.

Or do we crave foods that seem to take all our pain away, comfort us, make us feel safe for just a minute and send us into a sugar coma? What do we crave? We each have to answer that question honestly.

Here's what David said he craved. "One thing I crave from God, the one thing I seek above all else. I want the privilege of living with Him every moment in His house, finding the sweet loveliness of His face, filled with awe, delighting in His glory and grace. I want to live my life so close to Him that He takes pleasure in my every prayer."[9]

Paul gave this advice to the Galatians. "As you yield freely and fully to the dynamic life and power of the Holy Spirit, you will abandon the cravings of your self-life."[10]

Jesus said, "Bread alone will not satisfy, but true life is found in every word, which constantly goes forth from God's mouth."[11]

We need to be like David. We need to be like Paul. We need to be like Jesus.

QUESTIONS

1. What do you crave that you shouldn't? List those.

1.

2.

3.

4.

5.

2. What does God want you to crave? List those.

1.

2.

3.

4.

5.

3. Make a stop-start based on stopping some of the negative things you crave and starting to desire some of the things God wants you to crave. List it here.

4. In what ways are you prideful in the way you live your life? In the foods you eat? In the way you present yourself? In the weight you've lost?

5. If humility is total submission to God, are you a humble person? If not, what is holding you back from being humble? Do you desire to be humble? What is a stop-start you can make to begin to step into a more humble and God-submissive lifestyle?

(ENDNOTES)

1. James 4:1-10 NASB
2. James 4:1-10, Teresa Parker's personal application
3. Philippians 3:19 NIV
4. 1 Samuel 16:7 CEB
5. Matthew 23:12 TLB
6. Isaiah 57:15 NLT
7. Deuteronomy 8:2-3 NKJV
8. 3 John 2 AMP
9. Psalm 27:4 TPT
10. Galatians 5:16 TPT
11. Matthew 4:4 TPT

TRANSFORMATION FROM GLORY TO GLORY

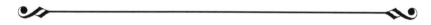

P lant an ugly old bulb in October and by spring it will transform into a beautiful tulip. Plant an acorn and it will transform into an oak tree, though it will take years to do so. Watch certain caterpillars and they will eventually transform into beautiful butterflies, one of the most glorious transformations on earth. These are natural transformations.

I'm a fan of transformation. That's why I love watching home remodeling shows. It settles my soul to watch Chip and Joanna of the television show *Fixer Upper* find an old, falling down shack on a perfect piece of land and use that to build a new house that becomes a beautiful, comfortable modern family home with antique farmhouse touches.

They had the vision to see what it could be and the owners were able to trust their vision enough to allow them to perform what seems like a miracle to those watching. These home remodeling shows reinforce my belief that transformation can happen to anything or anyone, even us.

TRANSFORMING FROM BIRTH

Transformation begins from the day we are born. By year one the tiny newborn weighing eight pounds will triple its birth weight. In the next year weight gain slows down. At the same time, the child is getting taller, learning new things and expanding its understanding of the world around him. In short, he is transforming in front of our eyes from a helpless child into a self-sufficient adult.

The dictionary definition of transformation is a complete change in someone or something's physical appearance or form. All of these examples fit this definition. The definition, though, doesn't really denote how long this process will take.

These days it's easier to keep up with the changes friends' children go through if we are friends through social media. I saw a picture of some friends I had seen recently, but hadn't seen their children. The last time I saw the kids they were toddlers. Looking at their photo it felt like they had transformed in a matter of minutes into high school graduates. Of course, it was years, but in my mind the time had flown by quickly.

MY TRANSFORMATION

In 2004 I weighed 430 lbs. By 2012 I had lost over 250 pounds. From where I was to where I am now fits the definition of physical transformation. I found that when I'd lost more than 150 pounds I began having to introduce myself to old friends or family I'd meet.

Recently my husband and I decided to go a restaurant we used to frequent, but hadn't been to in probably 10 years. It is close to our church and we used to eat there every Sunday until they closed on Sundays.

After we enjoyed the meal, Roy went to pay the bill as I was collecting my things to leave. The cashier is the wife of the owner. She used to check us out all those years ago. When I got up to the counter I found out she had asked Roy about his new wife.

All she remembered about me was my extreme size. She thought I was not the same woman Roy had been with before. I assured her I was the same person, just physically less of me. Upon thinking about it that really isn't true. I have transformed in more ways than just my physical appearance. It's just that the inner transformation may not be as visible as the outer.

CHANGE COMES FROM WITHIN

People look at the outward appearance, but God looks at the heart.[1] What did He see when He looked at mine? When I was super morbidly obese I thought my heart, which is the seat of my desires, was good but was it? I also thought my spiritual relationship with God was great, but was it?

The way we humans define transformation is by what we can see. Thus, a tulip, an oak tree, a butterfly, a high school graduate, a beautiful house, and someone who has lost an extreme amount of weight are pictures of transformation because we can see the change.

God, though, defines transformation differently. In the original Greek language, transformation is a change in form from one stage to the next in the life history of an organism, as from caterpillar to pupa and pupa to the adult butterfly.

In God's kingdom, though, in order to transform we must "fix our attention on God" in order to be "changed from the inside out."[2] Something has to happen on the inside to be able to transform completely. Then the results will be shown on the outside.

To transform we must "present our bodies, dedicating all of ourselves, set apart, as a living sacrifice, holy and well-pleasing to God, which is our rational, logical, intelligent act of worship."[3] Presenting our bodies as a living sacrifice means everything we think we want must be laid at the feet of Jesus.

We must think like Abraham when God told him to sacrifice his only son that he and his wife had prayed for and waited many years for. He had to be willing to lay him on the altar and kill him if necessary. This very act alone revealed the intent of Abraham's heart was to follow God and trust Him explicitly.

SURRENDERING ALL

For years I felt like sugar and high carbohydrate content foods were necessary for me to exist. They had become my go-to source for everything, but in order to transform from the inside out I chose to sacrifice or surrender them to God. I chose to do without.

When I made that decision, I started to be transformed and progressively changed as I began to really mature spiritually. I was finally allowing God to totally renew my mind by focusing on godly values and ethical attitudes instead of what I wanted.[4]

Once we do that something exciting happens. We are no longer just blindly walking through life. We have finally proven for ourselves what the will of God is for us. We are following Him with our eyes wide open.

The will of God is different for everyone. Things start to change when we decide that no matter what God asks of us we will do, even surrendering the foods we think of as rewards in this life.

Things become clearer and we finally begin to get a glimpse of what His plan and purpose is for us individually. We see that it truly is good, acceptable, and perfect because it was tailor-made for us.[5]

Understanding that surrendering completely to God is the way to discover His specific will for each one of us will help us to stop trying to fit into the ideals and opinions of the culture around us or of what we think we should become due to everyone else's expectations.

> Things start to change when we decide that no matter what God asks of us we will do, even surrendering the foods we think of as rewards in this life.

Then we will be inwardly transformed by the Holy Spirit through a total upheaval of how we view our life's purpose. This will empower us to discern God's will as we live beautiful lives, satisfying and perfect in His eyes.[6]

God desires that we be inwardly transformed by allowing the Holy Spirit to do a total reformation of what we think we should eat, when we should eat, and how much we should eat.

When we give up our dependence on foods that do not fuel our bodies and only fuel our selfish desires, only then can we live that beautiful life that is satisfying and perfect in His eyes.

SACRIFICING ISAAC

First, we have to sacrifice our Isaac. Our Isaac is that one thing we love more than God. We must kill our selfish desires. For many of us it feels like our personal stash of goodies is the only thing in this world that we have left to get us through the day.

Abraham was different from us. He had laid everything on the line for God. He left his homeland. He journeyed to a faraway land. The only thing he possessed that had the potential of meaning more to him than God was Isaac. God required that Abraham demonstrate his extreme love for Him because He had even greater things in mind for Abraham.

Down through the ages, the nation of Israel repeated Abraham's name over and over again. They served the God of Abraham, Isaac, and Jacob. All three of these men were very human and flawed, but they allowed God to work through them to get rid of the idols, or potential idols, in their lives.

I am very aware that I made my appetite for food an idol or a god in my life. It's difficult to admit, but it is more than true. I see it now, but I couldn't see it when I was in that habitually destructive lifestyle.

Paul minces no words warning us about this kind of lifestyle. "Stick with me, friends. Keep track of those you see running this same course, headed for this same goal. There are many out there taking other paths, choosing other goals, and trying to get you to go along with them. I've warned you of them many times; sadly, I'm having to do it again. All they want is easy street. They hate Christ's cross. But easy street is a dead-end street. Those who live there make their bellies their gods; belches are their praise; all they can think of is their appetites.

"But there's far more to life for us. We're citizens of high heaven. We're waiting the arrival of the Savior, the Master, Jesus Christ, who will transform our earthy bodies into glorious bodies like His own. He'll make us beautiful and whole with the same powerful skill by which He is putting everything as it should be, under and around Him."[7]

As a Wise Overcomer, I now know which foods will take me off my destiny course. If I start eating those foods again they will only harm me, not help me. That's why these verses are so important to me. I don't want to live a lifestyle that God sees as shameful. I look forward to total transformation when Jesus takes our humble bodies and transfigures us into the identical likeness of His glorified body.[8]

TOWARDS TRANSFORMATION

It will help us on our journeys if we remember that "we can all draw close to Him with the veil removed from our faces. And with no veil we all become like mirrors who brightly reflect the glory of the Lord Jesus, we are being transfigured or transformed into His very image as we move from one brighter level of glory to another, and this glorious transfiguration comes from the Lord, who is the Spirit."[9]

How does transformation happen? It happens as we move from glory to glory or as we go through the stages of transformation. As we move from Wishful Thinker to Wise

SWEET JOURNEY TO TRANSFORMATION

Overcomer "we grow into spiritual maturity both in mind and character, actively integrating godly values into our daily lives as our heavenly Father is perfect."[10]

As we live our lives, we go forward from the Wishful Thinker dreaming about what it would be like to change, to the Willing Owner who defines her issue and surrenders it to God, to the Watchful Learner who begins learning tools to help her start the transformation process, to the Wholehearted Traveler who actually begins to walk out the transformation journey, and finally to the Wise Overcomer who has learned how to live in perpetual transformation.

Jesus is calling us to transform and help others do the same.

Once we are at the Wise Overcomer stage, we can help bring others up through the stages of transformation. It is a cycle that must be repeated often until all are living in the state of being daily transformed.

Our journey to transformation continues as we learn ways to follow Him closer, living out our ever-increasingly transformed journeys. Always, though, our transformation is not for ourselves alone. It is also for others. As Jesus gave His life for us we must do the same for others.

Jesus is our role model. He told us, "In this world you will have trouble. But take heart! I have overcome the world."[11]

He is calling us to begin the process of overcoming our intense desire for more food than we need. He is calling us to transform and help others do the same. In order to do that we must be willing to continually be improving and developing an understanding of our issues.

We will never have arrived this side of heaven. We are just continuing to transform. This is a journey that never ends, but the beauty of it is that it only gets better as we allow Him to bring us into our destinies.

Then we will become "God's poetry, a recreated people who will fulfill the destiny He has given each of us for we are joined to Jesus, the Anointed One. Even before we were born, God planned in advance our destiny and the good works we would do to fulfill it."[12]

> Stepping into God's destiny for us becomes our reason to be on, and continue, this journey to transformation.

Stepping into God's destiny becomes our reason to be on, and continue, this journey. We fully understand and accept that our destinies do not lie in living like the rest of the world eating junk food, candy, desserts, and comfort foods. We have the desire to make something of our lives.

We have a desire to follow God in all things. We have a desire to know, really know, and understand that even though we are just like common clay jars, we carry a glorious treasure within us so that the extraordinary overflow of power from our lives will be seen as God's not ours.[13]

We have a desire to overcome the temptations and cravings that pull us all day long. We have a desire to be transformed from glory to glory.[14]

We are committed to staying in tune with God and what He wants for us. We are ready to step into His destiny dream for our lives.

QUESTIONS

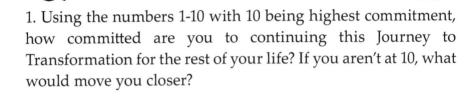

1. Using the numbers 1-10 with 10 being highest commitment, how committed are you to continuing this Journey to Transformation for the rest of your life? If you aren't at 10, what would move you closer?

2. What is your destiny dream?

3. What will you have to give up or stop in order to step into this destiny dream? When will you do this?

4. What will you have to start? When will you do this?

5. What will be your first step towards the transformation God has in mind for you? When will you take this first step?

(ENDNOTES)

1. 1 Samuel 16:7 NIV
2. Romans 12:2 MSG
3. Romans 12:1 AMP
4. Romans 12:2 AMP
5. Romans 12:1-2 MSG
6. Romans 12:2 TPT
7. Philippians 3: 17-21 MSG
8. Philippians 3:21 TPT
9. 2 Corinthians 3:17-18 TPT
10. Matthew 5:48 AMP
11. John 16:33 NIV
12. Ephesians 2:10 TPT
13. 2 Corinthians 4:7-8 TPT
14. 2 Corinthians 3:18 NIV

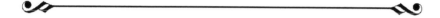

"We are convinced that every detail of our lives is continually woven together to fit into God's perfect plan of bringing good into our lives, for we are His lovers who have been called to fulfill His designed purpose."

Romans 8:28 TPT

MORE TESTIMONIES

My husband and I have been missionaries overseas for 47 years in a closed country. I am 72 years old and since age 13 I have been overweight. I've wanted to lose weight, but it seemed impossible for me.

I have lost 76 pounds and am keeping the weight off.

Then in 2016 I needed to lose weight in order to have a surgery. That same year my mother died after being unable to walk the last few years of her life. I didn't want to end our missionary time unable to walk. Finally, the Lord spoke clearly to me about losing weight.

By His leading I found Teresa's book, *Sweet Grace*. I really identified with her journey. Her coaching group was online, so I joined. In total, I have dropped over 76 pounds, walk more easily, and feel so much better. I finally understand how to lose weight and keep it off.

Jay Lee, Missionary to a Closed Country

WALKING THROUGH FOOD ADDICTION

I am so excited by where the Lord has taken me in this journey. I thought my issues were all about food. Walking through the lessons and letting Teresa guide me to bring down the barriers in my soul and life has been hard, but so beautiful.

I have found freedom and lost 43 pounds

My skewed thoughts of myself and food have kept me in a vicious cycle of destruction and failure for over 40 years. As God leads me through Teresa's teachings, ministering, and instructions, I am experiencing the healing in this area of food addiction.

I am now looking to God to discover the person He created me to be instead of trying to create that person is true freedom in Christ. I have found freedom and lost 43 pounds. I now know God has plans to prosper me and not to harm me!

Susan Keays, Whitehall, PA

TRANSFORMATION IS A LIFELONG PROCESS

I have struggled with weight all my life, going up and down over and over. The tools I have learned through Teresa's courses and coaching groups are helping to renew my mind. This applies in all areas of my life where I fail to depend on God and try to go it alone to "fix" me.

Transformation is a lifelong process. There are no quick fixes, just steady growth spiritually, mentally, emotionally, and physically. I thank God for all I have learned, the resulting changes in my life, and helping me lose 60 pounds.

Rhonda Burrows, Palestine, TX

LEARNING TO DEAL WITH MY EMOTIONS

I met Teresa over two years ago. Through her direction, I am finally learning how to deal with overeating and food addiction. She is the first person to help me deal with root issues that cause my overeating. Other weight loss groups put a bandaid over the problem and the weight always comes back.

Teresa believes that an intimate relationship with God is vital to recovery. She is showing me how to recognize and deal with emotions in a positive way instead of stuffing my feelings with food. I am learning to depend on God. Her lessons and coaching skills always point me back to Him.

Debbie Magner, Bradenton, FL

TURNING MY LIFE OVER TO JESUS

I read Teresa's book, *Sweet Grace,* and I felt like she was telling my story. I am 54 years old and I have been obese my whole life. I did all the commercial diets and had lap-band surgery. This still did not stop me from gaining weight.

I knew I was missing something. Teresa's book showed me that I can learn a new way of life. She led me to turn my life over to Jesus for the very first time. I'm learning how to trust Him for everything.

Now I can put the food down and live my life in the present. I do not have to do this program perfectly. I just have to be aware of my stops and starts and begin again. This is a lifestyle change journey and I am ready.

Sharon Temple, Yardville, NJ

HOPE FOR FOOD ADDICTION RECOVERY

The physical consequences of weighing close to a quarter of a ton for decades include existing in emotional despair and an agonizingly painful body.

In helplessness and despair, I cried out to God. He led me to Teresa's Holy Spirit-inspired books and lessons. They have helped me understand that my focus needs to be on my relationship with God and allowing Him to lead me with what and why I eat.

With 79 pounds gone, I now know how to go forward.

This was a totally new approach to losing weight. I recognized and accepted that I can do this. I gathered hope that freedom from my food addiction was not only possible, it was and is God's plan for me. I finally realized I am not beyond God's love and mercy.

Through time spent in deeper reflection, I began to see that my poor self-image made me feel unworthy of having good things, including a healthy body and the totality of God's love.

To date, I have lost 79 pounds. Though my health issues continue to be a daily struggle, I now know how to go forward. As long as I remain on earth my journey to transformation will continue.

It is my hope that God will be glorified through my journey and that as I continue to practice what I have learned and turn to God instead of food, He will be able to use my story to inspire others.

Lindy Brookhart Stevens, Valrico, FL

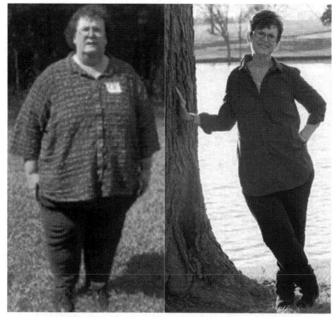

ABOUT THE AUTHOR

H i, I'm Teresa Shields Parker. Among other things, I'm an author, coach, and speaker. If you've read this book then you know I used to weigh 430 pounds and have lost over 250 pounds. Above, that's me in 2004 and me today.

I live in Columbia, MO with my husband, Roy, whom I'm still madly in love with even after 42 years of marriage. Our son, Andrew, and daughter, Jenny, and her husband, Nigel, all live in Columbia, as well.

Sweet Journey to Transformation is my fifth book. It is the seventh book in my Sweet Series, which also includes two study guides. My first book, *Sweet Grace: How I Lost 250 Pounds* has been number one in the Christian weight loss memoir category on Amazon for at least five years.

It was in January of 2013 when God clearly showed me I was to write my story of weight loss. I thought it would take me five years or longer to write a whole book. The book was written by June of 2013 and published in October of that year. By January of 2014 it had risen to number one in its category. For that to happen for a book from a first time self-published author was all God!

After people read the book, they wrote asking me to help them lose weight. I couldn't help them all individually so that's when God called me to form a Christian weight loss coaching group. That has mushroomed into other groups, courses, individual coaching, and even an Academy.

> I am passionate about helping Christians learn how to lose weight and transform.

This book actually began as one of my courses called Journey to Transformation. I now consider that my foundational course I am passionate about helping Christians learn how to begin to lose weight and transform—body, soul and spirit.

Diets do not provide lasting change. God's got a better way and part of that is dealing with issues that have held us back from stepping into all that He has for us. God can use anyone no matter what they weigh. However, I know that because of my weight I lacked the energy, clarity, focus, and passion I needed to live my calling.

I was eating my destiny every day. After I lost the weight and God called me to write my story, it felt like I finally stepped into exactly what I was created to do. However, it didn't happen until I lost weight.

Everywhere around me I see Christians who could be accomplishing much more if they just had the energy to do so. I now see clearly how I allowed the devil to steal my destiny for years and I want to help others caught in his trap.

My story is just one example of how God can use us at any age once we submit everything to Him, even what we eat and how we move. We can actually be a powerful force to be reckoned with when we get our weight under control.

After five years of coaching, I have a huge arsenal of teaching videos that have been used to set many free from excess weight and step into their personal transformations.

I decided to put these resources in an online vault and make it available for those willing to do the work. There are currently over 150 videos divided into over 21 courses. I'm calling this treasure chest, the Overcomers Academy.

Those who join the Academy also get access to a private Facebook group where my staff and I will be available to answer your questions. Journey to Transformation will be the featured course.

> My story is just one example of how God can use us at any age once we submit everything, even what we eat and how we move, to Him.

You've read the book and now I encourage you to join the Check out the Journey to Transformation course. Be sure to complete all the additional action steps and challenges available. Then dive into the rest of the courses to help you continue your journey.

In the private Facebook group you can meet others on the journey with you, post your victories and defeats, and support each other. My staff and I will be there cheering you on and answering your questions.

You've likely read the testimonies in this book. All of those folks have taken Journey to Transformation and many of the courses in the Academy.

> God called me to coach because I understand every excuse you have as to why you can't lose weight. I've had every one of them too.

You know my story and you know that I know what it feels like to be so overweight you feel you could die at any moment. I know what you're feeling. I even know what excuses you have as to why you can't lose weight. I've had every one of them too.

As a matter of fact, me understanding that was one reason I didn't want to be a coach. When I said that to God, He said, "That's exactly why I've called you to coach. You've been there and have come out. You're exactly the person to help them."

The only reason I do this is to help you connect more fully with God, who loves you and wants more than anything to see you prosper and be in good health.

I'm honored that you have read or are reading this book. If you need help putting these principles into action, check out the Academy, private coaching, or other helpful resources at www.TeresaShieldsParker.com.

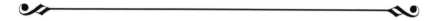

"As you yield freely and fully to the dynamic life and power of the Holy Spirit, you will abandon the cravings of your self-life."
Galatians 5:16 TPT

BOOKS BY TERESA SHIELDS PARKER

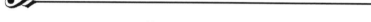

SWEET GRACE

Sweet Grace: How I Lost 250 Pounds and Stopped Trying To Earn God's Favor has been the #1 Christian weight loss memoir on Amazon since 2014. In it I chronicle my journey of walking out of sugar addiction by the grace and power of God.

I share honestly and transparently about what it is like to be super morbidly obese and what it takes to turn around and walk into food freedom.

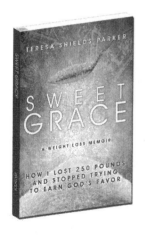

Get your copy in print, kindle or audiobook on Amazon. Add *Sweet Grace Study Guide: Practical Steps To Lose Weight And Overcome Sugar Addiction* to use in conjunction with *Sweet Grace* for personal or group study.

All of my books and study guides are also available for sale in .pdf format on my website.

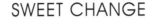

SWEET CHANGE

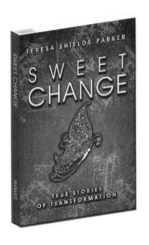

Sweet Change: True Stories of Transformation is all about the power of change and how to tap into it. I share stories of individuals who have found their own personal ingredients work great with God's power in order to lose weight and step into transformation. Get your copy on Amazon today.

SWEET FREEDOM

In *Sweet Freedom: Losing Weight and Keeping It Off With God's Help,* I walk you through my journey of dealing with emotional issues which kept me bound in sugar addiction for years. Almost anyone

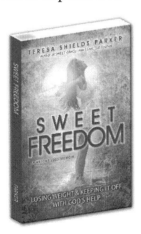

can lose weight, but most struggle and end up gaining it back again. I share my secrets to identifying and eradicating the emotional issues which became spiritual lies I began to allow to overwhelm me.

Get your copy in print, kindle or audiobook on Amazon. Don't forget *Sweet Freedom Study Guide,* which includes principles, concepts, tools and processes to help you on your journey to freedom from food addiction.

SWEET HUNGER

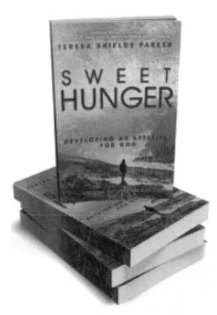

Sweet Hunger: Developing an Appetite for God is my first Bible study. In my own devotional time, I began to see how mentions of food in the Bible almost always coincide with God's presence.

Designed for personal Bible study, the eight lessons, questions and activities in the book can also be used for groups. Video teachings, along with a free downloadable Leader's Guide, are available at TeresaShieldsParker.com.

WEIGHT LOSS HELP AND OTHER RESOURCES

All my weight loss resources are on my website. This includes private coaching sessions called VIP Freedom Coaching, Overcomers Academy, and additional offers. Check under the Weight Loss tab for current resources. I also have many great items under my free tab on the website. I'm always adding and changing up things so check back often.

GO TO:

www.TeresaShieldsParker.com

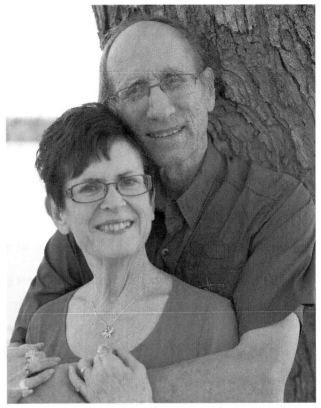

Teresa and Roy Parker

CONNECT WITH TERESA

WEBSITE: TeresaShieldsParker.com
EMAIL: Info@TeresaShieldsParker.com
FACEBOOK: Facebook.com/TeresaShieldsParker
Amazon: Amazon.com/author/TeresaShieldsParker/
Instagram: Instagram.com/treeparker
Twitter: Twitter.com/treeparker
Pinterest: Pinterest.com/treeparker

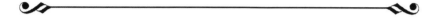

"Here's the one thing I crave from God,

the one thing I seek above all else:

I want the privilege of living with Him

every moment in His house."

Psalm 27:4 TPT

Made in the USA
Middletown, DE
01 May 2022